Beyond the Body

Death and social identity

Elizabeth Hallam, Jenny Hockey and Glennys Howarth

London and New York

First published 1999
by Routledge
11 New Fetter Lane, London EC4P 4EE

Simultaneously published in the USA and Canada
by Routledge
29 West 35th Street, New York, NY 10001

Routledge is an imprint of the Taylor & Francis Group

Typeset in Garamond by Routledge
Printed and bound in Great Britain by TJ International, Padstow, Cornwall

British Library Cataloguing in Publication Data
A catalogue record for this book is available from the British Library

Library of Congress Cataloging in Publication Data
A catalog record for this book has been requested

ISBN 0–415–18291–3 (hbk)
ISBN 0–415–18292–1 (pbk)

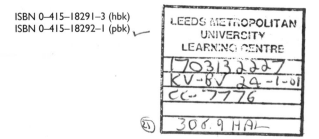

Contents

    Bibliography   211
    Index   222

Illustrations

Preface

This book came to life during the 2nd International Conference on Death, Dying and Disposal, held at the University of Sussex in 1996. This event brought the three of us together for the first time and led to a realisation that we shared similar interests in the body and death. We also shared a sense of frustration at the under-theorising of the body from within a death studies perspective. Furthermore, we were concerned at what appeared to be the trivialisation of death studies in theoretical approaches to mortality, and a neglect of the role of the dying or dead body in identity formation. For example, Bauman (1992) while lauding death studies as a now established field of social science research, is clear that his theoretical interests lie not with death but with the implications of mortality for the cultural strategies of life. Shilling also addresses death in his work on the body, but is at pains to point out that he is not concerned with death *per se*, but only with the effect that the encounter with death has on the embodied individual (1993: 203).

Our purpose in producing this text has been to engage in dialogues with some of these theoretical approaches to the body, and mortality. In contrast to Shilling, we would argue that the focus on embodied agency is inadequate in that it fails to take account of the ways in which meaning and identity can detach themselves from the living body. While the focus on embodied agency is significant, it marginalises those members of society who may be physically alive yet socially dead, and those biologically deceased who nevertheless retain an influential social presence in the lives of others. While socially dead bodies and disembodied selves seem to have been placed beyond the remit of a social theory of human embodiment and agency, this book argues that in failing to place disembodiment alongside embodiment, or to ask who or what is 'embodied' within the dementing or dying body, we are participating in the cultural and social processes which sequester death and dying. Rather than a social theory of the body which is limited by what are seen as the body's material boundaries, what we present here is an examination of human embodiment which situates itself at and beyond the body's boundaries. While we do not deny that social being and embodiment are intimately associated, we take the circumstances of death, in both a social and a biological sense, as our focus. In this way we develop our understanding of the implications of human materiality by exploring, rather than avoiding, situations which involve the dislocation of bodily and social being.

In considering the nature of a volume designed to address these issues we rejected the idea of producing an edited collection of snapshots of the dying or dead body and instead, made a conscious choice to co-author a text which deals directly with what we believed to be the more pressing theoretical issues outlined above. Thus, this work represents an integrated, jointly written examination of the book's core theoretical questions. Our work is informed by an historical and cross-cultural perspective but its primary agenda is pursued within the context of contemporary Western society. We are not, therefore, offering a continuous historical account of the social positioning of the dead body, nor do we provide an exhaustive review of death ritual in other societies.

Our disciplinary backgrounds encompass both historical and social anthropology, the sociology of health and the sociology of deviance. We share common interests in gender issues and, as the location of our first meeting discloses, a concern with the study of death and dying. We therefore brought to this project a diversity of theoretical and substantive issues which have been drawn together to critically examine the question of how the deteriorating, dying and dead body might be theorised. The volume draws on historical and cross-cultural material relating to the organisation of the dying and dead body by health professionals, morticians, coroners, church courts; to the ways in which clergy and clairvoyants access, and lay claim to control over the dead, and to ways in which surviving spouses may incorporate the dead into their lives. Some of the chapters draw on data from our own fieldwork or research. Chapter 3 employs field data from a study of a local authority residential home for older people. Chapter 5 is based on field research into the work of coroners and conducted in three geographical regions:

northern England, western England and London. Chapter 6 utilises material from the Canterbury Cathedral Archives and Library, Canterbury Archdeaconry and Consistory Court Depositions, 1580–1640. Chapter 7 uses data from an ethnographic study of funeral directors in the East End of London. Chapter 8 draws from a range of field studies conducted in a variety of locations, focusing primarily on qualitative interviews with elderly people and observations within a residential home. Chapter 9 also uses qualitative methods to consider the work of a Christian minister in Yorkshire in 1996. Chapter 10 relies on data from fieldwork with women who practised as clairvoyants in the Midlands, England.

Just as data has been drawn from a number of sources, so the collaborative writing which has resulted in this book was undertaken in a number of sites. The proposal began to take shape during the first, and a subsequent, meeting at the University of Sussex. From there we met together at a Cultural Studies Conference in Leeds, and then at the 3rd Social Context of Death, Dying and Disposal conference in Cardiff. Our first substantive periods of work on the text itself were undertaken in Durham, where Douglas Davies kindly hosted us in University accommodation and Bob Simpson found us a convenient and quiet workspace. We also worked in our own universities: Jenny in Hull, Liz initially at Sussex and then in Aberdeen, and Glennys, originally at Sussex and then across the world in Sydney, Australia. The book further developed at meetings in Manchester, Whitby, Edinburgh, Sheffield and Sydney. When the 4th Social Context of Death conference came around we found ourselves together again and working in Glasgow – our thanks to Margaret Mitchell for kindly lending us her home for three days at the end of the conference.

A number of other people have helped us with this project. We would especially like to thank: Louise Bourdua, Roy Boyne, Fidelma Farley, Ronnie Frankenberg, Steve Gallery, Mike Hepworth, Carol Komaromy, Ian MacLachlan, Bob Simpson and Deborah Wickering. Andrew Dawson and Mark Johnson provided stimulating comments during a 'kitchen table' seminar in Hull. Colleagues at the University of Aberdeen are thanked for helpful comments on the material presented in Chapter 2. Thanks also to colleagues at the University of Surrey for comments on an early version of Chapter 6.

LIZ HALLAM, JENNY HOCKEY AND GLENNYS HOWARTH, NOVEMBER 1998

Chapter 1

'Vegetables', 'vampires' and other hybrids

This book has been written within the context of developing social theories of the body.[1] These are theories which have acknowledged the centrality of the body in the formation of social identity but have as yet to pay sufficient attention to the dying and dead body. While sociologies have re-mapped the body in social and cultural terms, marginalised, problematic bodies remain a more peripheral focus of theoretical interest. Here we are pressing for an analysis of bodies in crisis which are undergoing radical transformation during crucial phases of the life course – and in particular, for attention to be paid to the formation of identity throughout the process of dying, at the point of, and after death. We argue that these bodies are experienced, interpreted and located in different ways with regard to social and cultural practices which are central to the constitution of self and other.

Central to the arguments advanced in this book is the view that the relationship between the body and the self may not be as straightforward as much of the existing sociological and anthropological work assumes. Not all bodies are synonymous with a self and not all selves have an embodied corporeal presence. For example, some individuals become categorised as 'just vegetables', a product of social practices and discourses which, in shaping the self in relation to the body in death, produce forms of social exclusion. On the other hand, the concept of beings such as 'vampires' indicate the possibility of a continued social presence for disembodied persons. Both 'vegetables' and 'vampires' are hybrids in that they confuse the cultural categories of life and death; they represent the dissolution of boundaries which organise key phases of the life course. They also fail to realise the relationship between body and self which is imagined within current social theories of the body; a relationship which is predicated upon the conflation of self and body. With reference to European cultural forms, Stallybrass and White define hybridisation as a 'mixing of binary opposites...such that there is a heterodox merging of elements usually perceived as incompatible [which] unsettles any fixed binaryism' (1986: 44). Thus, those identified as 'vegetables' and 'vampires' are perceived as unstable, dangerous and marginal within dominant social and cultural orders.

Throughout this book we attend to these excluded and marginalised social groups, focusing on bodily crises, instabilities and transformations associated with death and impinging in significant ways upon social identities. To this end, we begin by exploring the processes through which some individuals become metaphorically transformed into vegetables. This often arises from a combination of perceived physical ageing and mental confusion, which leads to the exclusion of individuals from social membership or participation. We also examine the continued social presence of disembodied individuals who have died. These are often recognised in exoticised forms – for example, ghosts, ancestors, revenants or vampires – beings which exist, from an orthodox perspective, on the deathly margins of society. Here we set disembodiment alongside embodiment in order to question our 'common-sense' assumption that selves necessarily reside within discrete bounded bodies. Unlike 'vegetables' which, in their social death (Mulkay, 1993) are regulated – stored away, or warehoused, within institutions (Miller and Gwynne, 1972), the biologically dead cannot necessarily be contained with such ease. They are potentially problematic for members of many societies and ethnographic accounts document the cultural and social strategies through which they may be managed, accessed or relocated. For example, gypsy dead are pinned down in the non-gypsy space of the Christian churchyard for fear that they will otherwise return to haunt their nomadic kin (Okely, 1983). Also, rural Greek dead become the pivot of a sequence of ritual practices which quite literally spiral around the body so that the soul will make an auspicious progression to its allotted place in another world which is profoundly different and indeed opposed to the world of the living. Neglect of these rituals brings the inauspicious return of the dead in the form of the vampire who drains the life-blood of the living while they are asleep (Du Boulay, 1982). In a similar vein, the focus of much Christian liturgy is the deliverance of the soul of the dead into the hands of God. As we show in Chapter 9, some Christian clergy recognise the possibility of problematic or failed passage to a heavenly sphere in that the dead may return to finish their life's incomplete projects.

Through its subject matter, therefore this volume attends to gaps in a matrix of body/selves which can be divided as follows:

socially and biologically alive : socially and biologically dead

socially dead/biologically alive : socially alive/biologically dead.

The first of the two pairs are privileged, both by the social sciences and indeed within everyday institutional discourses and practices. If we believe that life and death stand in a clear oppositional relationship to one another, then we expect to move across a binary opposition from being socially and biologically alive to being socially and biologically dead. Certain Western social ideals suggest that those who are physically alive are fully incorporated within society, if necessary receiving its support when they can no longer contribute to it. And once dead, while there may be an extended period of respectful remembrance, the deceased cannot and indeed should not be seen to participate in society. Recognised as society's living members, it is those with living bodies who can be seen to participate in the face-to-face encounters of 'everyday life', who represent the privileged focus of the sociological or anthropological gaze.

Here we focus on the socially dead/biologically alive: socially alive/biologically dead pairing. Both of these are hybrids and as such they evoke fear. To be terminally ill yet not extinguished is a fate dreaded by many and epitomised most poignantly in the individual with advanced Alzheimer's disease. Their relatives may grieve their loss, or social death, years before their bodies are eventually disposed of. Jonathan Miller, President of the Alzheimer's Disease Society, depicts Alzheimer's as a living death:

> when I talk to public meetings about it, I talk about it as an uncollected corpse, there is this terrible thing which is walking around, which the undertaker has cruelly forgotten to collect. Oh, I'm frightened of it. Yes, I am frightened.
>
> (1990: 230)

However, to remain socially alive after bodily demise can be similarly disruptive. It raises the spectre of the 'pathologically' grieving individual who enshrines their dead loved one and refuses to engage with the living. It also hints at ghosts, ancestors and spirits, which, from dominant Western perspectives, are often identified as features of 'other societies' or as manifestations of 'irrationality'. Thus, the notions of the living 'death' of dementia and the 'living' dead within our loneliness and nightmares, are predicated upon a social self which has become separated off from the physical body. This process is both fragile and dangerous. Not only are self and body differentiated from one another; they are also re-conjugated in illegitimate pairings.

This book is located among these shadowed conjugations: socially dead but biologically alive and socially alive but biologically dead. It asks what we might mean by social death and indeed what the possibility of social life after death might imply. By addressing these questions we problematise the ease with which 'life' and 'death' come to be differentiated from one another in such a definitive and exclusive a fashion.

Body becoming self

In 1982 Featherstone identified the twentieth century emergence of the 'performing self' where 'appearance, gesture and bodily demeanour become taken as expressions of self' (1991: 189). This and related perspectives on the body were drawn together by Shilling in 1993 when he argued that, 'in the conditions of high modernity, there is a tendency for the body to become increasingly central to the modern person's sense of self-identity' (1993: 1). These arguments stress the elision of body and self, highlighting 'penalties' exacted upon those whose bodies fail to live up to consumerist imagery, ageing, unkempt or disabled individuals can become socially dispossessed, if not 'dead' (Mulkay, 1993).

While social priorities attach themselves to young, healthy, sexually attractive bodies, therefore, it is readily assumed that those with less than perfect bodies have a lesser social presence. During the nineteenth century, self-improvement could be achieved through the development of 'character' forming habits. In contrast, twentieth century individuals are entreated by consumerist culture to develop their 'personalities', most crucially through the bodily resources of voice control, public speaking, exercise, 'healthy' eating, a good complexion, grooming and beauty aids (Featherstone, 1991: 188). This re-formulation of self ideal does, however, produce a 'self' which ultimately is extinguishable (Mulkay, 1993), with the result that embodied social identity is felt to come under serious threat through processes such as institutional ageing, hospital death and the management of the corpse by funeral directors, coroners and clergy.

For many social anthropologists, the time of death and its attendant ritual are seen as a key episode within the life of any particular society, the time and space within which core social values are represented, often in over-determined forms (see for example, Lévi-Strauss, 1973). Indeed, as Hertz argued in 1907, 'when a man dies, society loses in him much more than a unit; it is stricken in the very principle of its life, in the faith it has in itself' (1960: 78). Geertz similarly notes that death and its rituals not only reflect social values but also shape them in important ways (Huntington and Metcalf, 1979: 5). If, as social theorists contend, the body is a key site within which the self is realised, arguably, it is precisely towards the period of its deterioration and disposal that we should train our eye. For example, it is then that the self as constituted across time begins a radical process of transformation. Diachronically unfolding biographies collapse and condense in parting reconciliations, eulogies, reminiscence, graveside relationships and the gathering and subsequent dispersal of anecdotes, clothing and memorabilia. Holistically and synchronically, fragments of personal identity may be gathered, sifted and recast. That which is left unsaid or unexpressed, those entire identities which prove irrecoverable, constitute disturbing silences which resonate powerfully within a society where the biographical continuity of the individual is afforded high priority (Giddens, 1991: 54).

The body in death highlights the passage of time, the inevitability of physical transformation, and thereby acts as a powerful reminder that the self is subject to change. Furthermore, the conceptual frameworks through which this transforming self comes to be understood, are also constituted within dynamic social and cultural relations. Bodies have personal histories, and these are always emergent within longer-term historical processes. Thus Porter points to a complex of 'religious, moral and value systems' which change over time to construe various relationships between body, mind and soul; between disorderly bodies and disciplinary regimes; between individual bodies, communities, and the wider body politic (1991). The body is always located within historically specific discourses and practices which formulate and connect the inner and outer body in different ways. With reference to contemporary Western society, Turner notes that through technologies such as photography, the ageing body is recorded and reflected upon. But as there is difficulty in acknowledging the ageing process, there emerges 'a necessary disjuncture between the inner self and the image of the body' (1995: 250). The ways in which the body in decline and death are conceived in relation to the self are, therefore, shaped in important ways by historically emergent cultural representations.

Theorising the body

In seeking to reconcile the polarities of the body as either a natural, pre-social entity amenable to cultural and social elaboration or the product of discourse, knowable only through discourse, Shilling has described it as 'an entity which is in the process of becoming' (1993). He identifies a finishing process which encompasses the changes which the body undergoes over time – for example, the imprint of habitual facial expressions and bodily postures upon flesh and skeleton. The precise nature of these physical changes, of course, reflects social and cultural influences – for example, specific bodily styles, or techniques (Mauss, 1973 [1934]); socially structured material resources such as diet or housing; and the professional practices of medicine. Giddens (1991) argues for a distinctively Western 'finishing' of the body which involves more than just adherence to cultural styles or traditional practices such as body decoration. Rather, it is the outcome of a reflexive process whereby the body, as a resource, is made to contribute to the production of a consciously chosen social identity. Though varying in degree from cosmetic surgery to choice of hairstyle, Giddens none the less insists that members of Western societies cannot act outside of an awareness of the diversity of identities which surround them (1991: 70–108). This extends into everyday choices and practices. For example, the selection of particular food stuffs from a diverse range of alternative possibilities, rather than the reproduction of an inevitable pattern of consumption.

Shilling's desire to reconcile naturalistic and constructionist accounts of the body produces an account which requires social constructionists to engage with the body's materiality (1993: 12–13). And in the realm of social constructionism, we find a division among sociologists which is often recognised in shorthand form as the agency/structure debate. Thus the accounts of theorists such as Goffman (1959), Featherstone and Hepworth (1991) and Giddens (1991) privilege the individual's agency, their ability to manage the body in particular ways in face-to-face interactions. It is thus, in the view of these theorists, that the individual participates in society. This foregrounding of action, control and agency as a means to frame embodiment reflects one of sociology's traditional interests – in society as (inter-)action, event and process. The body is therefore a resource to be mobilised or capital to be safeguarded and exploited, albeit within particular sets of constraints, identified variously as biological, social or structural. This reflexive engagement with body projects is, however, an approach which cannot easily account for the embodied experience of those whose bodies have become extremely frail and/or brain function has diminished.

Conversely, debate which draws on a Foucauldian perspective, such as the earlier work of Bryan Turner (1984), offers an account of the body as the product of discourse, an entity which has no *a priori* existence but rather comes into being through a micro-politics of power targeted at the regulation of the flesh and the production of the docile body. While accounts of the body which take its agency as a starting point may not always provide very satisfactory accounts of the intersection of individual agency with macro-level structures, those which focus on the influence of discourses which are external to the individual provide less insight into the phenomenology of embodied social life. That is to say, they give little space to the grounded, sensual experience of inhabiting a body. This limitation becomes particularly evident when bodies which are old and frail are the focus. When older women and men become subject to discourses surrounding a concept such as 'social death', we are left without the necessary theoretical apparatus to discuss the nature of their subjectivities.

The notion of embodiment, or embodied human agency (Giddens, 1991), provides a bridge between materialist and discursive perspectives and here we draw upon Thomas Csordas' work in this area (1994). His critique of the privileging of representation or discourse highlights problems such as the linked assumption that subjectivity is internally located, a source of representations which are then projected upon an outside world. In its place he sets a model of subjectivity as 'interpersonal engage-ment via a "conversational" form within a world constituted by existential concerns' (1994: 9). In other words, he suggests that our subjectivities are inter-subjective, that they are constituted within the existential spaces which link and divide us from one another. Csordas moves on to discuss anthropological critiques of representation which, for example, argue that it subjugates the bodily to the semantic (Jackson, cited in Csordas, 1994: 10). Seeking a term which can more adequately capture the existential immediacy which so often escapes work focused on representation, he suggests 'being-in-the-world' (ibid.). This, he argues, allows for a focus on 'temporally/historically informed sensory presence and engagement' (ibid.). He also critiques a view of language as a form of discourse without which we cannot 'know' our own embodied experience. Drawing on the work of Paul Ricoeur, he suggests that 'language gives access to a world of experience in so far as experience comes to, or is brought to, language' (ibid.: 11). Language is therefore another modality of being-in-the-world.

The intersubjective self

Throughout this book, we approach human embodiment in relation to forms of human disembodiment. We would argue that to neglect the analysis of bodies in crisis is to participate in the sequestration of death and dying. Rather, we need to problematise a cultural ethos where independence and control are valorised at the expense of intimacy and surrender. The current focus on embodiment, to the exclusion of disembodiment, perhaps reflects the notion that the death of the body means that the individual has ceased to be. Indeed, should an individual become extremely frail or confused prior to biological death, we may even feel that they have already died before the point at which their body finally expires. This easy conflation of individual and body requires interrogation. For instance, it fails to account adequately for the ways in which cultural meanings and social identities are assigned to both the foetus and the corpse, neither of which have the capacity to act independently; it also fails to account for the ways in which meaning and identity can 'detach' themselves from the living body. In its place we need to develop an understanding of how, or if, the 'life' of someone with dementia or someone who is 'brain dead' on a life support system may be constituted, both culturally and socially. We also need to question the elision of embodiment, agency and social identity, and raise questions about its implications for those members of society who have a profoundly vital and influential social presence, yet who lack a living body – be they ancestors, martyrs or dead children; a reference in an archive, a corpse in preparation for disposal; or a 'voice' brought into being by a clairvoyant.

Csordas posits embodiment as 'an indeterminate methodological field defined by perceptual experience and mode of presence and engagement in the world', something which is akin to the phenomenological notion of intersubjectivity (1994: 12). It is this focus on a shared, dialogic physicality which sits uneasily with a notion of embodied agency expressed in the autonomous, body-based construction of self-identity – through, for example, fitness regimes, patterns of consumption, and sexual practices (for example, Featherstone, [1991] 1995; Grosz and Probyn, 1995). Here, cross-cultural comparisons are useful in highlighting and problematising dominant Western conceptions. From Fiji, Becker provides an example of agency as a collective phenomenon, where 'bodily experience transcends the individual body, is diffused to other bodies, and is even manifest in the environment' (1995: 127). Theirs is a society in which an abundance of food is highly prized, yet corpulent bodies reflect not the status or competence of the individual, but rather the collectivity's ability to nurture and care for its members. As Becker notes, 'the self...while certainly connected to its body, is not its exclusive agent'. For Becker, therefore, like Csordas, embodied experience is 'contingent on how the self is situated in a relational matrix' (1994: 127). While Becker makes a straightforward comparison between the Western unity of the individualised body/self and the collectivity of Fijian embodiment, she does, however, gloss over the differences which together constitute that Western experience. In effect, her characterisation of the Western experience of embodiment rests upon an assumption that it is produced, universally, by the metaphor of the body as a container (Johnson, cited in Battersby, 1993). Writing from within Western culture, Battersby, on the other hand, takes issue with the universality of this experience; when confronted with this model of the body, she states, 'I register a shock of strangeness: of wondering what it would be like to inhabit a body like that' (1993: 31). As a feminist, Battersby argues that Western models of self-identity privilege 'form, solidity, optics and fixity' (1993: 34), at the cost of fluidity, a notion of self permeated by otherness. In this alternative model of self 'the boundary between the inside and the outside, between self and not-self, has to operate not antagonistically –

according to the logic of containment – but in terms of patterns of flow' (ibid.: 35). She argues that the experience of embodiment as an intersubjective process has existed alongside a more patriarchal focus on containment and exclusion. Indeed, she suggests that the containment which seems to characterise patriarchal thought and experience should itself be viewed as but one feature within a wider process of change.

Battersby's work is significant in identifying the limitations and particularity of the embodied, individualised agency which is seen to characterise Western experience. She foregrounds other voices, other bodies, other experiences of self. And it is within this possibility of an alternative, marginalised relationship between self and body that we here locate the dead and dying body, arguing that it forces a vital awareness of the partiality of concepts such as agency, embodiment and self-identity as they are currently understood. While there has recently been a call for a reformulation of what is meant by corporeality, this endeavour often bows out at the point at which the body features most vividly, if painfully, within human consciousness – during the time of disease, distress or dysfunction. As Csordas points out, in everyday experience the body often 'disappears' – as opposed to the sense of alienation or absence from one's body which is experienced during pain or disability. Indeed, he goes on to cite Leenhardt's work on the pre-objective and objectified body, showing that among the New Caledonian Peoples with whom he was working, the body was not individuated, either from the spirit or from other individuals, but instead 'diffused with other persons and things in a unitary sociomythic domain' (1994: 7). In other words it was pre-objectified. Only through representational forms and practices such as colonial Christianity, biological science or consumer culture do the perceptual processes of the body result in objectification (ibid.). Chapter 2 in this volume makes central this question of how representation might shape, and be shaped by, experiences of the body. The objectification of the body is also addressed by Becker, again with respect to illness and pain, where 'as a locus of pain, the body takes on agency over and against the self' (Good, cited in Becker, 1995: 31). Thus in distress the individual may feel alienated from their body. In the place of its 'unreflective harmony' (Zegans, cited in Becker, 1995: 31), the body begins to 'invade' the individual's thoughts (Murphy, cited in Becker, 1995:31). Not only is the objectified body experienced as a separate, distanced entity, but also, in different circumstances, as a trap which inhibits the inner self. For example, a 'thin' person may feel trapped inside a 'fat' body, or with regard to gender – a 'woman' might feel trapped inside a 'man's' body (ibid.: 32).

In much of the social theory of the body, however, the issues of death and dying, if not illness, still require further examination. At present we struggle with the question of who or what is 'embodied' within the dementing or dying body (Lawton, 1998); and we are disturbed by the ongoing social presence of individuals who are dead. Indeed, those whose daily lives continue to be lived out in what they regard as intimate proximity to deceased partners or children, have, until recently, been diagnosed as suffering from 'pathological grief'. It is only in the 1990s that work such as Klass et al.'s Continuing Bonds (1996) has provided an acknowledgement of the pervasiveness of the disembodied social presence of the dead, both historically and within contemporary social relationships. As Simpson argues, the realm of 'imagined' social relationships has hitherto been seen as the province of psychologists and psychoanalysts, a separation which reflects a distinction between inner 'private' and external 'social' realities. Drawing on Bakhtin's notion of dialogical constructions (1981), Simpson notes that, 'the imagined world itself is populated with characters "felt to be there" which continually splice into the real world' (1998).

Once we have engaged with accounts of different cultures, we are better placed to recognise a deeper and more complex sociality which often characterises social relationships. Becker, for example, explores a lack of synchrony between body and self in Fiji, arguing that, 'the two, body and self, do not share a mutually fixed or exclusive identity; their common substrate is the collective' (1995: 127). Yet dominant within contemporary theories of the body is an ethos within which the body is imaged as the finite container of a self defined primarily in terms of its separation from other bodies. This, we argue, is a highly localised reading of the body and its role in identity construction. In its place stands the need for a new theoretical stance which situates itself at and beyond the body's material boundaries, so engaging with those who have no body or who are nobody. As Battersby argues, 'the boundary of my body should rather be thought of as an event-horizon, in which one form (myself) meets its potentiality for transforming itself into another form or forms (the not-self)' (1993: 36).

Destabilising dichotomies

In the following chapters we develop the agenda outlined so far, focusing on material drawn largely from historical and contemporary Britain. The relationships between embodied experience and cultural representations are explored in Chapter 2 where we make visual representation a starting point in examining historically and socially specific experiences of the body in crisis. In the chapters which follow from this, we move from the ageing and dying body to the dead body and its management and interpretation. Finally, in Chapters 8, 9 and 10, we shift our attention 'beyond the body' in an examination of the continued social presence of the dead. Incorporating examples of ethnographic and archival research conducted both by the authors of this book and others, this chronological progression from dying to death and departure might seem a self-evident structure if we wish to examine the human body at the edge of life, through death and after disposal. However, one of our central tasks is to question the assumed opposition between 'life' and 'death' which is characteristic of contemporary Western societies. Although we follow what might seem to be a 'natural', biologically grounded pathway from life to death, our aim is to destabilise many of its associated empirical and theoretical binaries: body and mind; inner body and outer body; self and other; corpse and spirit; magic and science; pre-modern and modern; illusion and reality; fixity and process; connection and disconnection; proximity and distance. Each of these dichotomies is, we argue, an historically emergent, cultural construct. As we develop our argument, these are examined through a range of case studies, together with ethnographic and archival examples. For death, as Prior (1989) has shown, has been experienced and interpreted in a variety of quite particular, context specific ways; for example, through institutionalised classificatory systems such as public health. And indeed, as this book will show, although the body in and after death has been the object of a range of dominant discourses – legal, medical, religious – it is experienced both between and across these discourses. When viewed from a local perspective, therefore, the relationships between life and death and the body and self emerge as far more fluid and variable than when seen from a macro-level view which represents them as a highly dichotomised set of relationships. Death, as we shall see, is everywhere encoded in life and life is encoded in death in a complex, self-referential relationship. As Bronfen and Goodwin

argue, 'Just as the theoretical lines drawn between binary oppositions have been coming under fire, so the actual – living and
breathing – boundary between life and death has become a matter
of urgent debate, for both ends of the life cycle' (1993: 5–6). Jenks
(1998) invites sociologists to approach their subject matter through
dichotomous thinking, arguing that it opens up the possibility of a
more active engagement with difference or the middle ground. It is
precisely this invitation which we have taken up in the writing of
this book.

Our starting point for examining the body in crisis as a problematic site for social identity is the old body as it deteriorates and dies.
Using data gathered during the 1980s within a residential home for
older adults in the North East of England, we show that in this
context, strategies of distancing and control served to rob people of
an individuality which may have become troubling for both families
and carers (Hockey, 1990). The result is that the older person's
disease or infirmity often remains as the single marker of self. This
attrition of personal identity can produce an elision between old age
and poor health, with the result that illnesses both chronic and
acute become naturalised as aspects of later life. However, while for
an outsider the 'self' becomes subsumed within the condition, for
older people themselves the self may actually come to be experienced as separable from the condition and indeed from the body
itself. As Chapter 3 suggests, individuals may come to relate to
their bodies from a variety of positions in later life, a situation
which produces the possibility of multiple bodies and multiple
selves.

Theoretical work on the old and/or sick body offers competing
approaches to data of this kind. Csordas (1994) and Becker (1995)
characterise illness as an experience of the body as ungovernable;
something which can produce objectifications. The individual then
either distances themselves from a troubling physicality, or acts
purposefully upon their own body. This process is acknowledged in
Featherstone and Hepworth's concept of the 'mask of ageing'. The
metaphor of the mask conveys the sense of alienation experienced by
older people when an 'inauthentic' identity which they do not
recognise or experience at first hand is none the less read off from
their wrinkled, bent, shuffling bodies (1991).

In contrast Shilling's notion of the unfinished body which
becomes, as described by Illich 'a progressive embodiment of self'
(Illich, cited in Becker, 1995), suggests that later life embodiment

might, if anything, be a more marked and profound experience of the body than in earlier life. Carrying a layering, indeed sedimentation of social thought and action, the old body is a project which can require the individual's continuous application or agency. Field data from the study cited above reveal the vigour and tenacity of residents' embodied self-identity (Hockey, 1990).

A further example of the complex relationship between self-identity and body is revealed in an analysis of the medical treatment of the stillborn infant and the adult in a persistent vegetative state. Here we see hybrids produced as the binary relationship or differentiation between 'life' and 'death' becomes even more radically destabilised. Previously categorised within hospitals as a yet-to-become human entity or indeed as waste, organic matter, to be disposed of in an unmarked grave, the assignment of social identity to the stillborn body is established, and for some, institutionalised in social hospital-generated practices such as cuddling, dressing, naming, photographing and funerary ritual. In this way a 'daughter' or 'son' is produced (Heald with Brown, 1994; Hockey, 1996; Lovell, 1997). Conversely, the 'life-like' appearance of the 'brain dead' body stubbornly sustains a pre-existing set of social relations. For relatives, the persistence of the comatose individual's previous social identity can make the switching-off of a ventilator and the surgical removal of an organ an act of killing, followed by a violation of the body (Robbins, 1996).

In both these cases, the status of the dead body as a material object which somehow contains the 'truth' or 'reality' of 'death' has been problematised. Lay and professional discourses together produce a multiplicity of 'bodies' and 'deaths'. While the social identity of the stillborn body derives entirely from its imagined future, the comatose body sustains a past and present self which is very much 'alive' to those around them. Unlike older adults in residential care, these two categories of body have died while firmly located within the context of social life and as such they can remain socially alive, whether in the immediate past or the anticipated future.

The ambiguities which surround death in the womb or on a life support machine often reproduce themselves in the case of sudden death. In the coroner's court, professional and lay constructions of the biography of the deceased individual are produced. While the examples already cited involve the reconstruction and projection of the social identity of the deceased into the future, responses to sudden death mean that the body becomes a starting point for a retrospective narrative reconstruction of a person's former life. The pathologist explores the surfaces of the body and examines the internal organs in order to locate it in time and space, pinpointing the moment of death and its physiological causes. As the object of their professional gaze, this body bears a history: a medical history read via scar tissue, lesions and damaged organs; and a social history, accessed via tattoos, body piercing, clothing and other objects found on or around the body. Thus, during the inquest, coroners struggle with relatives, friends, work mates, pathologists and institutional representatives to recreate a social being which is recognisable to all. However, for the coroner, pathologist and other professionals, the corpse is an objective source of knowledge; while for bereaved people it is not simply a body but a person. Seeking to understand the death, relatives draw on experts' reports, in combination with their own, more intimate knowledge of the deceased's body, to locate the death within an ongoing biography.

The task of identity construction through the medium of the corpse is also shouldered by those professionals who undertake the management of the dead body. Data from an ethnographic study of funeral directors show that their first encounter with the body is usually in death (Howarth, 1996). Through their practice and their language, funeral directors and embalmers distance themselves from a now stigmatised cadaver, while simultaneously seeking to humanise it. Profane, yet sacred to bereaved family and friends and a site for meaningful relationships with the living, the corpse is prepared by morticians who employ the language of identity and personality, projecting desires such as clothing choice and hairstyle onto their subjects. Striving to produce a body which closely resembles the living body remembered by survivors, funeral directors recreate the order so often destroyed by the illness or violence which led to the death. Embalmers apply their skills to remove signs of damage: wounds are cleaned, sealed and hidden; discoloration is expunged with transfusions of formaldehyde; facial expressions which indicate trauma are smoothed, eyes closed, lips sealed. The memory picture presented to mourners who come to view the deceased is intended to reveal a state of well-being, present in the body they recognise as belonging to the person in life. In this way, funeral directors and their staff play a key role in fulfilling many bereaved people's need to prolong meaningful contact with the body of the deceased.

The example of funeral directors' practices around, within and upon the surface of the corpse, exemplifies the ways in which the dead body can be made to represent the individual associated with it. However, in the absence of the body, social presence may still persist and it is this continuity which most radically challenges the current sociological claims that we become social beings only through our embodiment. Though studies suggest that older bereaved people are vulnerable to social isolation (Mulkay and Ernst, 1991), data indicate that many continue to enjoy significant social relationships with their 'dead' spouse. Rather than the materiality of the body, clothing and significant sounds, sights and smells associated with the former partner begin to assume powerful, new resonances. Although such resonances are often perceived by rationally minded sociologists to be an illusion or delusion, we would argue that such relationships merit more serious consideration in that they destabilise the modern dualism which separates the worlds of the living and the dead.

Alongside the practices of funeral directors, can be placed the work of Christian ministers. The Christian Church has exercised a profound influence upon the way in which relationships between earthly and spiritual domains are construed. Ariès has observed that:

> the fact that life has an end is not overlooked, but this end never coincides with physical death. It depends on the unknown state of the beyond, the solidity or ephemerality of survival, the persistence of memory, the erosion of fame, and the intervention of supernatural beings.
>
> ([1977] 1983: 64)

Alongside a prevailing willingness to hope for, if not believe in, some kind of post-mortal social identity, the Christian Church intervenes in a highly ambiguous relationship which links many members of Western societies with the dead. Though the liturgical practices of the funeral service are concerned with the relocation of the dead and the re-ordering of relationships between survivors, the requirement to 'let go' of the dead is often unrealised. Instead the dead find their way into the everyday lives of those who survive them. Dead children 'grow up' via the birthday celebrations of their parents, and dead parents, in turn, continue to shape the lives of their surviving children (Riches and Dawson, 1997). At times the dead become 'embodied' through the materialisation of a spirit or 'ghost' (Finucane, 1996).

Positioned as Other in relation to the living, such disembodied beings are perceived to be both troubled and troubling. Data which document the work of a contemporary minister, well known for his skills in exorcism, suggest that such beings are viewed as matter out of place which can only be re-positioned through the prayers and ritual practices of the Church – and also as a challenge to the current limitations of scientific knowledge (Hockey, 1999). In his account, the minister frames the experience of haunting within sets of scientific metaphors. These, we suggest, fulfil two purposes. As explanations for these phenomena, scientific metaphors constitute a resource through which an attempt can be made to order or domesticate them. However, an additional and contradictory strategy is apparent in that these metaphors also contribute to the 'othering' of the apparitions, flying objects, unaccountable sounds and nauseating smells which he describes. In that science is popularly thought of as 'logical', 'rational' and 'objective', it is felt to stand outside the messy 'subjectivity' of everyday common-sense understandings. In being so distanced, science acquires a mystique as a body of arcane, almost magical knowledge. As such, it provides a rhetorical device through which to heighten, even dramatise, the non-ordinariness of the materialised dead. However, although firmly located as separate and Other, the dead are also illegitimate in their continued social presence within the lives of their survivors. Clergy therefore feel that, in the case of a haunting, the relocation of the dead which, in their view is completed at the time of the funeral, must, in these special cases, be re-attempted. It is with an expert voice of power and authority that clergy bid the dead to move forward into their rightful places. Although widespread, the fear of haunting reflects a complex set of social contradictions in that ours is an environment where the dead are both called back by bereaved individuals, yet kept at a distance within institutionalised religion.

As noted, Ariès has signposted the variety of sources and sites which may shape the ending of life ([1977] 1983). If we wish to unpick the privileging of the body within contemporary construc-tions of social identity, the area of magical beliefs and practices can provide us with important insights into selective imaginings associated with corporeality. For example, research among informal ritual specialists such as clairvoyants show that their practices are underpinned by epistemological assumptions which challenge mainstream, positivist models of the material – or corporeal – world and its limits (Hallam, 1997b). Although their beliefs and practices are often constructed as erroneous, corrupt or clandestine, clairvoyants' encounters with clients can be crucial in the reconstitution of self and identity at points of crisis such as death. Underlying their orientation towards the disincarnate, lies a different figuring of the boundary between the living body and those who have gone before. With the use of various ritualised techniques, clairvoyants manage life/death crises through 'readings' of the client's body and their spiritual attendants.

Drawing on the studies detailed above, this book enters the debates spawned by a critique of traditional sociology – that it leaves the body out of its frame. Turner points out that in 1984, when *The Body and Society* was published, apart from work which drew on Foucauldian perspectives, 'there was little interest in mainstream social sciences and humanities in the sociology of the body' (1996: 1). In the present volume, we argue that this more recent recovery of the body is distinctly partial. The current sociology of the body may help us make sense of the corporeal lives of some of society's members; but it excludes many others, namely those at the margins or those at the edge of life. We have chosen to focus on the creatures of the margins by putting the 'vegetables' and the 'vampires' among us at centre stage. We suggest that the omission of the disembodied self from social theories of the body mirrors the beliefs and practices of dominant social groups and institutions which disavow the continued social presence or participation of the dead.

Among recent social theories of the body a particular view of human agency is foregrounded. It is expressed most typically in the post-traditional project of self-construction (Giddens, 1991). In the conditions of high modernity, we catch the embodied self at work, free to reconstitute itself along the lines of its own choice, but adrift among the competing influences of fashion, science, medicine and the media. As this book will argue, agency, expressed in reconstructive tasks such as health care, fitness regimes and plastic surgery, can be seen merely as the individual resisting the body's constraints and limitations in a spurious attempt to deflect awareness of its inevitably mortal nature (Bauman, 1992). Thus, while the gendered body, the medicalised body, the consumer body and the fit body have been fruitful areas for study, authors literally exhaust their material in that all such bodies are simultaneously in the process of ageing and dying. It is this theoretical orientation which has led us to question whether the dying and dead body can be encompassed within a social theory which foregrounds embodiment in analyses of human agency. For example, Shilling, in his book *The Body and Social Theory* addresses the implications of the dead body for those whose bodies are alive. As he points out, however, 'my interest...was less on the dead body, though, and more on the embodied individual's confrontation with death' (1993: 203).

One of the reasons for these exclusions, we suggest, is that rather than the self experienced via agency and the tasks of self-construction, the body in crisis appears to undermine the individual's capacity for self-mobilisation in relation to a surrounding environment. It is a state of affairs which invites the spectre of the constructed rather than constructing self and so carries a particular threat for an academic community which still retains something of its capacity for self-determination. However, as we argue, social theory is underpinned by a set of assumptions about embodied agency which often overlook the intersubjective and indeed collective nature of self-identity, not only in life but also in death. For bereaved individuals, for funeral directors, embalmers, coroners, solicitors and the clergy, the corpse, the grave, the will and the empty armchair can form powerful evocations of full-bodied if absent persons. The academic community may have identified embodied agency as its focus in a necessary curb on earlier theorising which saw the mind as the seat of social being and the body as merely its container and its object. But in its present form this concept offers limited explanatory capacity with regard to the precise relationship between, on the one hand, human embodiment and, on the other, social identity. In this re-examination of the fate of the dying and dead body we challenge the view that the self inevitably founders with the dissolution of the container-body. As Battersby argues 'not all talk of identity involves thinking of the self as unitary or contained; nor indeed need boundaries be conceived in ways that make the identity closed, autonomous or impermeable' (1993: 38).

Note
[1] See Nettleton (1998) for a critical summary of this work.

Chapter 2

The dying body

Visual representations

The role of cultural representations within perceptions and experiences of the dying and dead body remains a subject of debate both within anthropological and sociological studies and within the wider contemporary public domain. This chapter addresses the ways in which the dying, dead and decaying body has been viewed, interpreted and assigned social and moral meanings via a range of visual forms including printed images, material objects, films and photographs. This leads to questions regarding the ways in which representations of the dead and dying body operate within the social and cultural processes which constitute selves, including those of the dying and deceased. Bronfen claims that 'One cannot speak of an "essential" self preceding the social and cultural construction of self through the agency of representations' (Bronfen, 1992: 65). The dying, dead and decaying body has formed a compelling focus of Western European visual cultures, such that an exploration of the cultural construction of corporeality demands an analysis of visual forms such as these. Attending to the nuanced meanings of visual representations of the dead body requires an appreciation of cultural and historical context: the ways in which such images were produced and deployed within wider discourses and practices which shape perceptions of the self, personal morality, spirituality, conduct and social order. This chapter is concerned with the range of meanings encoded within such images, paying particular attention to the ways in which they work to construct notions of self and social identity.

Within social theories of the body, the socio-cultural construction and presentation of the self are increasingly understood as complex processes within which embodiment plays a crucial role. In modern societies bodily appearance, action and gesture are recognised through social interaction as expressions of the self

(Featherstone, [1991] 1995: 189). While the body and, therefore the self, can be styled in a variety of ways within consumer culture, a certain degree of self-analysis and reflexivity is required to achieve this. Turner suggests that self-reflexivity is particularly apparent during phases of the life course when the body is subject to change. So for example the ageing of the body may act as a stimulus for reflexivity and furthermore, he argues 'the aging of generations and the aging of individuals becomes intensely problematic since the emphasis on activism and individualism must necessarily conflict with the inevitable biological decay of the individual self' (Turner, 1995, 258). Self-reflection thus becomes more pronounced when the limits of the physical body are experienced.

Evidence examined in the later chapters of this book suggests that the body in crisis, especially in death, forms a site at which notions of self and social identity are highlighted. As we shall see, witnessing or experiencing the body in decline through death or decay forms a potent reminder of frailty, vulnerability and mortality. The passage of time and the inevitability of physical transformation become powerfully evident. They provoke anxieties about the integrity of the body as it faces destruction. When emphasis is placed upon control and the regulation of the body as a prerequisite for the maintenance of self-identity, the dying body and the dead body acquire terrifying qualities. These bodies render visible the processes which are denied in the pursuit of an ideal which rests upon the control of bodily boundaries; for example, the passage of organic matter out of the body, the management of movement in limbs and facial muscles.

The individualising of self

In Chapter 1 we introduced debates about the nature of the self, indicating that contemporary models, both popular and academic, are highly specific to contemporary Western society. Asad (1998) identifies the seventeenth century as the period during which religious imperatives to save one's 'self' and Cartesian models of mind, or consciousness, as separable from the body together contributed to the formation of an individuated self or subject. Ariès, in his work on death states that there was an important relationship between an awareness of self or individuality and attitudes to death (Ariès, [1977] 1983). This issue has also been explored with reference to early modern death ritual where Gittings argues that the individuality of the deceased and a concern for only their immediate family was ritually marked through monuments and mourning dress. She claims that:

> [t]he anxiety which resulted from growing individualism is revealed in a desire to separate the living and the dead, and in an increasing horror at the idea of physical decomposition, as shown, for example by the growth in the use of coffins at burials.
>
> (Gittings, 1984: 102)

These arguments suggest that from the early modern period onwards death began to be displaced, in association with the emergence of a particular sense of self, and manifested most significantly in the disposal of the corpse in funerary ritual. Ariès notes, the corpse was covered in the 'successive masks' of the shroud, and the coffin, eventually to become a 'theatrical monument' (Ariès, [1977] 1983: 607). We might note, however, that the elaboration of the cultural devices used to conceal the body in death, actually worked to draw the eye towards it.

Recent historical work, addressing the medieval and early modern periods, has emphasised the significance of visual culture in the formation of attitudes towards death, in the ritualised practices surrounding this life crisis and in the production of ideas about the body (Llewellyn, 1991; Camille, 1994; Binski, 1996). The analysis of visual culture in these accounts addresses a broad domain of relics, altar pieces, printed images, paintings, monuments, memorials and tombs, funeral effigies, mourning objects and attire. The cultural elaboration of the dying and dead body in visual terms therefore developed as a highly charged process invested with religious, social, political and personal significance. However, Camille notes a tendency in historical studies to prioritise a 'reading' of the body based on textual sources. Working against this textual paradigm he foregrounds the visual image in the articulation of ideas about the body which worked to construct communal and individual identities during the Middle Ages (Camille, 1994). These historical studies of death imagery, when set alongside analyses of contemporary visual cultures, embracing film (especially horror genres), photography and museum displays, highlight the cultural potency of the visual in the shaping of embodied experience. What is suggested by this complex and extensive domain of images devoted to the visible rendering of the body in decline, is that there is, however historically variable, a cultural apparatus which recovers the disappearing body. Operating through various media and continuing to resonate over time, there has been a proliferation of imagery centring on the dying body which effectively maintains its social presence.

These issues are particularly pertinent in relation to dying and dead bodies in that they have been removed, in varying degrees, from the direct gaze and replaced with sophisticated systems of representation. With reference to Elias' work, Featherstone and Wernick highlight a resistance to the acknowledgement of 'bodily decline' (1995: 2) which would mark a cultural retreat from visual experiences of death. Ruby identifies a related transformation of 'real' death into 'fictionalized' images through contemporary media. The proliferation of representations of death serves only to reinforce our distance from it: 'Our culture is permeated by images and accounts of death, but they are only fictions, works of imagination, counterfeits. The real thing is carefully hidden.' (Lesy, 1987: 3–4, quoted in Ruby, 1995: 12). Although we may talk of a denial or a disappearance of death, a focus on the role of visual representations reveals more complex processes at work. Moreover, these are processes which operate in a variety of ways and reflect a diversity of social, moral and political agendas.

Representing the 'real'

In engaging with the role of representation, we encounter important questions concerning the relation of representation to what is conceived of as the 'real' dying and dead body. The relationships between imaged death, on the one hand, and embodied death, on the other, are construed in complex ways which are culturally and historically variable. With reference to images and texts from the eighteenth century onwards, Bronfen discusses the relationships between the represented body and the concrete physicality of dying: 'what is intensely real to the dying body is intensely unreal to the spectator of this dying body' (Bronfen, 1992: 45). While the process of another's death might be closely observed, the state of death can only be approximated: 'death as a state can rightly be regarded not as something which is sometimes represented, but rather as something which can only be represented' (Binski, 1996: 70). For the experience of dying to be communicated it must be translated from the realm of the private into a 'public world of signs'. Yet there is always a sense in which representations cannot adequately convey the reality of this experience. As Bronfen argues further:

> [t]ransforming the real body experience of death into an objectified form mitigates the violence posed by the real. Hence such a transformation can be seen as a personal or cultural strategy of self-preservation. The threat that real death poses to any sense of stability, wholeness, individual uniqueness or immortality is antidoted through representations that 'exteriorize' this real by transferring it on to an image/signifier.
>
> (Bronfen, 1992: 46)

The process of representation referred to here is therefore one which allows the dying and dead body to be made visible, yet at the same time functions to mask the material reality of embodied death and its destabilising effects. The radical disorder invoked by the dying and decaying body is countered by representations which 'fix' this process in the form of an image. The work of representation in this respect aspires to, but, in Bronfen's analysis, ultimately fails to 'counteract the destruction of a stable construction of self, which is called forth by an experience of the violence of death' (ibid.: 53).

> Provoking the spectator or reader to hover between denial and acknowledgement, narrative representations of death (whether visual or textual) serve to show that any 'voyeur' is always also implicated in the field of vision and that the act of fragmenting and objectifying the body of another ricochets back by destabilising the spectator's position as well.
>
> (ibid.: 54)

The viewing of representations of the dying and dead body would therefore appear to heighten self-reflexivity. The contemplation of the self in relation to images of another's death, depending in part upon the capacity of this imagery to implicate the viewer, has occurred in a variety of historical contexts which are explored below. Despite the apparent 'otherness' of the body in death, and the extent to which representations have become 'fictionalised', they retain a potency which provides them with significance in the cultural formation of self and social identity. The interplay of presence and absence which renders the dying body and the body after death visible, and therefore active in social life, has been negotiated through a variety of cultural devices and technologies. These are introduced in this chapter beginning with an examination of medieval and early modern cultural forms and extending into a consideration of nineteenth and twentieth century representations.

Shifting visualities

Acknowledging the role of visual cultures in the formation of ideas about the body in death, and related concepts of self, entails not only an analysis of visual images and material objects, but also an examination of the cultural assumptions which underpin visuality. The boundaries between the visible and the invisible shift over time since the gaze itself, as well as the objects available for visual contemplation, are historically and culturally produced. The realm of visibility is culturally delineated and the viewing positions available within any given visual field are shaped in crucial ways by cultural codes, social relations and practices (Jay, 1996). Relationships between spectator and image are complex, given that a multiplicity of interpretations might be derived from a single image and that their meanings are likely to shift over time. In addition, representations are produced, used and circulated in a variety of ways. Mellor and Shilling note that much of contemporary sociological analysis of the body has focused on representations and images. However, they identify problems in this approach:

> (w)hile analyses of the discursive or textual construction of bodies tell us much about how the body is seen and portrayed, they usually fail to account for what it is about the body that allows it to be depicted and constructed in certain ways, or why the body has become such a popular object of representation.
>
> (Mellor and Shilling, 1997: 5)

In outlining the limitations of a theoretical focus on representations, they note, for instance, that factors such as human agency and the lived experience of the body are neglected. They propose to move beyond the study of representations through an emphasis on the body not just as an 'object of sociological investigation, but as an inherently sociological and historical phenomenon' with important sensory experiences (ibid.: 5). They argue that while vision is prioritised in contemporary Western culture and, indeed equated with access to knowledge, the epistemological bases of the other senses should be recognised as socially and culturally significant. The emphasis on sight as the primary sensual process which mediates the body's relation to knowledge should be understood as a culturally and historically specific orientation. As Mellor and Shilling point out: '[t]he postmodern concern with images and representations itself reflects what Jenks (1995: 7) has called "a serious commitment to surface", whose corresponding commitment to the visual has obliterated any sense of the body's ontological depth' (1997: 26). At stake here are the ways in which visual representations and embodied experiences are related. How are the surfaces of the body and the inner self formulated and connected via cultural representation? Here we argue that analysis of visual representations is crucial if we are to understand how embodiment is shaped. Social and cultural perspectives on the body in death cannot be developed without an account of the significance of representations.

Viewing bodies: an historical perspective

Responses to images of the dying and dead body can be powerfully ambivalent. At once fascinating and repulsive, such images variously associate the body with notions about the social, the sacred, the political and the erotic, depending upon their positioning within wider image repertoires and historical contexts. In anthropological analysis these issues have been discussed in terms of bodily, social and conceptual boundaries (Douglas, 1966). While our focus is visual representations *of* the body, we also acknowledge anthropological work which explores the body *as* a system of representation.

The body itself has been conceptualised as a potent symbolic resource which has the capacity to represent wider cultural notions about the individual and society, order and disorder, power and spirituality. Douglas's influential analysis of symbolic boundaries explores the significance of the body as a source of symbolism for complex social structures. In social contexts where the body and its related parts are used in ritual practices to represent aspects of the social system, Douglas notes that bodily margins or boundaries are 'specially invested with power and danger' (Douglas, [1966] 1988: 121). Boundaries are the points at which the bodily (and by association social) structures are particularly vulnerable. Bodily dirt and waste, which has transgressed these boundaries is often imbued with creative or destructive powers. Douglas is therefore able to cite, for example, the ritual use of the Lovedu queen's remains in attempts to control the material environment (ibid.: 120). Her decaying corpse is used to make unguents which her successor employs to control the weather. The corpse is, here, used in a ritual system which defends the social group faced by threats to its well-being. The corpse on one level becomes dirty and polluting as its bodily boundaries are no longer controllable, dissolving in the process of decay. The transgression of bodily boundaries is dangerous as it confuses the inside and the outside of the body. But with this sense of danger comes power which can be manipulated in ritual contexts to uphold the social structure. Thus Douglas describes a cultural logic through which the unclean becomes sacred, and therefore powerful and fascinating. This logic can be seen at work in the Western context where medieval images of the crucifixion display Christ's dying body as a source of sacred power.

A further argument developed by Stallybrass and White (1986) would account for the intersection of revulsion and fascination associated with the body in death. With reference to Northern Europe from the sixteenth century onwards, they describe the transformation of certain cultural forms and their associated concepts of the body. They highlight a shift away from the grotesque body, which was celebrated in medieval popular festivals, and a movement towards the classical body which was associated with the high, official culture of the Renaissance. The grotesque body, found at the centre of carnivals, prioritised the fleshy, material aspects of life: food, sex and violence. Most significantly it was a body in process, in that all of the bodily orifices were open and so its limits were not clearly defined. The grotesque body celebrated all bodily processes including birth and death and so expressed a particular folk conception of the body as part of a festive cycle of life and renewal; death was not feared but was embraced and trans-formed through the grotesque body and its symbolism.

Stallybrass and White, drawing on the work of Bakhtin, show how the grotesque body was progressively marginalised by the rise of the classical body (1986). The classical body, represented in Renaissance statues, was a static body with clearly defined boundaries. It was smooth, controlled and elevated on plinths. This model of the controlled, individual body was increasingly favoured by rising middle class groups who defined the grotesque body as offensive to bourgeois sensibilities. The grotesque, a body which embraced death, was therefore defined as contaminating, dirty and threatening. The consolidation of the classical body as the dominant model marginalised and excluded the grotesque and this process was central to the formation of a middle-class identity which rested on the cleanliness and control of the body. The dying body, with its messy confusion and unstable boundaries, had no place within this dominant model.

The cultural exclusion of the grotesque body was, however, never completed. While the middle classes defined it as disgusting and sought to push it out of the public domain, it remained a source of fascination and resurfaced in nineteenth and twentieth century cultural forms – such as art and literature. Thus Stallybrass and White propose that 'disgust always bears the imprint of desire' (1986: 191). The bodily processes rejected by the bourgeois sensibility remained, by virtue of their offensive and threatening nature, a source of fascination. This deep ambivalence can therefore be noted as an important aspect of the European cultural politics of the body. As Bronfen observes with reference to images of the dying body: they mask, or 'conceal what is too dangerous to articulate openly but too fascinating to repress successfully' (1992, xi). Her point is consistent with Ariès' argument that, as death becomes remote within European culture, it remains fascinating – arousing curiosity and forming a source of fantasy (Ariès, [1977] 1983: 608).

As the work of these authors indicates, the location of the corpse, its distance or proximity, both at the level of social practice and at the level of representation has been negotiated through a complex field of cultural devices. This chapter argues that the distancing or masking of death, and the concepts of the body that this worked to construct, was not a simple linear process. It is evident that what is construed as the reality of death is often brought powerfully before the eyes. And even when images of the body in death are deployed as a metaphor, they retain a powerful influence within social, spiritual and political relations. We move on, now, to look more closely at how perceptions of the dying and dead body have shifted across time.

Turner asserts that through modernisation we have witnessed the 'emergence of somatic society, that is, a society in which the problems of the body dominate the centre stage of political debate and political process' (1995: 258). While Turner highlights the centrality of the body within late twentieth century practices and discourses, he also identifies the body as a deeply embedded historical concern when he suggests that 'the body has always been problematised by the cultural legacies of Christianity' (ibid.: 256). It is useful, here, to trace some significant features of medieval and early modern conceptions of the dead and dying body with particular reference to the visual dimensions of these constructs.

Camille notes that during the medieval period 'the human body was the site of intense visual scrutiny and surveillance by the Church' (1994: 62). Within medieval Christian thought, notions about the body were organised around two sets of conflicting ideas: the body formed a site of impurity and corruption but at the same time it was a site of the holy and incorruptible (Binski, 1996: 70). The medieval person was composed of a body and a soul, progressively moving through transformative crises, like baptism and death, in a process determined by God. The dead were not to be feared; instead relationships between the living and the dead were carefully maintained. From the point of death, Christian souls would enter purgatory where they were cleansed of sins before their passage into Heaven. This process was aided by the prayers of the living who, therefore, had direct responsibility for the afterlife of the dead.

Binski argues that Christianity effectively 'demarginalised' the dead, creating closer links between the living and the deceased through a variety of means. Christian belief in saints, who had ascended to Heaven but remained physically present on earth through relics or fragments of their physical bodies, ensured that the worlds of the living and the dead were increasingly mediated at shrines (Binski, 1996: 11–14). Binski also identifies an epistemological shift whereby sensual experience was reorganised, so that the faculty of sight was prioritised as a means of accessing the holy dead. Previously there had been an emphasis on touch as the point of contact between saints relics and those seeking their healing effect. By the twelfth century, shrines were fully elevated within churches to form potent visual displays of saints' bodies which were perceived to be active and effective in healing the sick (ibid.: 78). By the fourteenth century the visualising of Christ's suffering, dying body was also central to religious experience; for example, images of the crucifixion centre upon Christ's suffering body as a positive means to salvation.

The dead and the living were also brought into conjunction at the site of tombs where the dead were displayed in the form of three-dimensional effigies. Here the instability of their flesh was removed from the gaze as the natural body, prone to decay, was replaced by a static image of the dead in a stable, idealised state. The dead body was taken out of time and represented as simultaneously deceased and life-like. Effigies functioned to display a person's social status, conveyed through their dress and therefore linked the physical body to the wider body politic, maintaining hierarchies of rank and power. They also constructed notions of selfhood, conceived in terms of a person's particular position within a system of social groupings. Such representations retained the social presence of the dead and marked out their identity primarily in terms of their association with lineage and kinship ties, their position within ecclesiastical hierarchies or their occupation.

The development of macabre imagery brought representations of the dead further into view within medieval visual culture, particularly after the Black Death. Between the twelfth and the fifteenth centuries death itself was personified in the form of a cadaver. Death was rendered as active and triumphant, circulating at every level of society to transform it. Three main forms of the macabre emerged during this period. Firstly, images of the Three Living and Three Dead depicts three hunters in a forest, who encounter three corpses in various stages of decomposition. The living and the dead enter into a dialogue in which the dead advise the living to improve their ways, to reflect on their mortal condition and to remember the transience of life. The dead therefore point to the nature of the human condition and through a process of 'shock, fascination and self-realization' the living receive moral instruction (Binski, 1996: 134). The imaged dead trigger self-contemplation in the imaged living and thereby invite the viewer of the image to enter into personal reflection.

The second form of the macabre, the transi tomb, also provided a visual means which allowed particular models of the relationship between body and the self to be displayed. Laid one above the other, the two bodies of the transi tomb represented the dead as both a social and a natural body. The dead appeared as a body, but with their social position and rank intact. Beneath them lay their 'body double', rendered as a corpse, naked and stripped of signs of social participation (Figure 1). The body in decay represented the inner sinfulness of the body and the viewer was invited to contemplate the fate of their bodies through inscriptions which typically proclaimed 'you who will be like me after you die: horrible in all things, dust, worms, vile flesh' (Binski, 1996: 143). Binski argues that the transi tomb was a form of anti-representation in that it challenged or destabilised the effigy which had previously replaced the natural decaying body with the idealised social body. The effigy had served to distance decomposition, but the transi tomb exposed this illusion. In this sense it 'performed a kind of unmasking of that which had hitherto been concealed' (ibid.: 149). The transi tomb thus revealed the fate of the flesh, but did so as a means to inspire spiritual and moral reflection in the viewer.

The third form of the macabre, images of the dance of death, also operated as a powerful reminder of death. The central theme was the notion that everyone, regardless of rank would face death (Illich, 1976). Death is shown as an animated skeleton circulating freely amongst the living. Death is triumphant in that everyone must succumb to its invitation (Figure 2). These images operate, on one level, to collapse the social hierarchy in that members of every group are drawn into death's dance (see Watt, 1994 [1991]. But they also displayed the distinctions between social groups, and therefore reinforced social and political inequalities. The Dance of Death also alludes to vice and the corruption of the flesh as dance was associated with sensuality and seduction. So here again, images of death offer a commentary on the condition of the living and invite contemplation of the self in relation to the social, moral and spiritual order.

These macabre images were regarded as mirrors of mortality and were referred to as such in contemporary sermons and manuals of religious instruction. They reflected the truth about a person's present and inevitable future condition. The mirror can therefore provide an instrument which intensifies self-reflection, forming an aid to self-understanding. Mirrors of mortality mobilised images of the dead body to shape the inner condition of the living. They also functioned to define social difference, including gender difference.

The convention of the mirror points to the significance of visual perception in the medieval culture of death. Yet there was a critique of excessive curiosity in that the 'lust of the eye' was regarded as a source of sin closely related to the 'lust of the flesh'. Here there are significant gender dimensions which worked through a variety of visual representations mobilising images of death which extended into the sixteenth and seventeenth centuries. Women were regarded as particularly prone to both the lust of the eye and of the flesh. For example in sixteenth century printed images, women are criticised for their excessive vanity and pride with regard to their bodies. *The Description of Pride* (1569) is based on a story from a manual of

religious instruction which described a woman who sent her maid
out to buy a looking glass. The maid returned with a skull which,
she declared, is the best mirror in which to see yourself (Figure 3).
The message is clear, the woman should not be concerned with her
surface appearance, but should contemplate the inevitable fate of
her flesh and therefore her inner spiritual condition. In a seventeenth century version of *The Mirror of Life and Death*, women were
warned that their physical beauty was only temporary. Woman
becomes a hybrid creature, half-life and half-death, a fertile living
body but also a dead and decaying form. The cultural associations
between women and death ran deeply through these representations
and found their source in the Garden of Eden where Eve's fall from
grace introduced human mortality (Borin, 1993).

There were connections between sin, self-knowledge and death in
the Christian tradition which were far-reaching in structuring
relations between women and men. Eve, open to temptation by the
devil, transgresses, and is therefore directly linked to the dangers of
the flesh, disorderly sexuality and death. These connections are
made visible in *The Tree of Knowledge and Death* (1587) which shows
Eve as the root of man's downfall and links her sin with death
(Figure 4) (see Hallam, 1997a: 111). These images appropriate
elements of the macabre (the mirror, the cadaver) and deploy them
in moralising commentaries directed against women. Death
highlights the corruption of women's flesh, mocks their preoccupation with surface appearances and inverts the association of the
female body and birth. Material of this kind exemplifies the
complex agendas which are brought into play via the 'viewing of
bodies'. Here visual representations of death serve to reinforce
gender hierarchies among the living. In addition, the mirror of
death was also used in critiques of earthly hierarchies of power. Even
the highest in the land could be brought down by death. *The Mirror
which Flatters Not* (Carey, 1639), held up by the king in deathly
form, was printed just prior to the English civil war, thus marking
the transitory nature of power (Figure 5).

Printed images of this type were intended to comment upon and
to shape public conduct and morality. They were circulated widely
and aimed to instruct the spiritual community, both in life and
death. Images of the deathbed were particularly significant in this
respect. Such images guided the preparation of the dying for their
final moments, preparations which were also important in the
maintenance of reputation and status (Hallam, 1996). As a result,

cleanliness and the management of the dying body through ritualised gestures and prayers, were crucial. Deathbed practices were informed and structured by codes of conduct which were reproduced and disseminated through the church and 'official', as well as popular, illustrated texts (Figure 6).

Images of the deathbed were intended to instruct and therefore to shape embodied practices: the successful art of death was comprised of interrelated images, physical gestures and sentiments sanctioned by the church and wider spiritual community (see Cressy, 1997). Together with the rituals with which they were associated, images of death carried moralising messages which conveyed ideas about the virtues, duties, and modes of conduct required in the maintenance of social 'credit' or reputation among the living. Therefore the social evaluation of a person's life was intimately bound to their display of a 'good' death. Rather than a system of representation which isolated death from life, here we see images of death used to inform both the living and the dying as to appropriate spiritual conduct. This, in turn, was something which impacted on their social reputation in life.

The simultaneous presence of a living body and dead body was therefore constantly reiterated in the early modern iconography of death. Portraits embraced the living and the dead body within the same representational space; love, marriage and symbols of the beginning of life being visually located alongside death. The presence of death, or a culturally articulated awareness of mortality, within everyday life was further evidenced in the extended and ritualised process of dying which could extend for years prior to the actual moment of death. We argue, therefore, that if we assume a clear binary opposition between life and death, we will be unable to make sense of the way relationships between the living and the dead were conceived of during the early modern period: 'Post-Reformation emblematic images...are, however, intended to present life and death as part of a single cultural process, not as opposing values in a crude binary model of the human condition' (Llewellyn, 1991: 10). Yet despite material of this kind, processual models of a continuity between life and death, where both states impinge upon and shape the other, still remain relatively unexplored within current social theories of embodiment.

To sum up the key issues which emerge from discussion of this historical period, we need to note that images of the body were produced in the context of religious devotion and ritual. The ritual disposal of the corpse removed it from the direct gaze and it was replaced by a range of representations which effectively preserved the social presence of the dead. Such representations maintained close relationships between the living and the dead and linked the bodies of the living and those of the dead into a wider spiritual framework. These images were intended to move the living towards a deeper self-understanding and to prepare the dying for the afterlife, for their rebirth. The images also worked to uphold spiritual and social hierarchies and offered commentaries on the moral condition of the living. Representations of this type constituted differences between bodies: the sacred and the powerful, the morally upright and the sinful. But they also formed a potent means by which the individual body was linked to collective social and spiritual bodies. And just as these representations of the body reinforced social hierarchies, they could also be used to challenge them. The metaphor of bodily decay, decomposition and disorder was a potent device in the criticism of social and political order.

Viewing bodies: contemporary issues

Townsend observes that the 'radical change of the twentieth century has been the effacement of death from public and wider familial experience. Death's representation, except through fantasized, cinematic violence, has largely disappeared from Western culture' (1998: 131). He accounts for this change largely in terms of the emergence of a perceived dichotomy between life and death, a separation which defines death as 'other' and marks a divergence from early modern conceptions of life and death as a continuous process. Thus Townsend highlights the dominant perception that death and the dying body are located at and beyond the margins of society. His discussion overlooks the fact that from the mid-nineteenth century to the present day visual images of the dead have been generated and deployed through a range of cultural practices. While analysis of the social uses of death imagery has emphasised their limited accessibility (Townsend, 1998), we would argue that their potency in terms of shaping self-identities and experiences of embodiment have been underestimated. Turner proposes that 'our embodiment is crucial, not only to our understanding of our most fundamental existential experiences such as birth and death, but also to an appreciation of basic processes such as memory and identity' (1995: 251). Furthermore, the development of photography and other technological means by which images of the body are preserved and displayed, for example, video and film, has been significant in the shaping of memories of the body and its transformations over time. When analysed in the context of the institutional sites and social interactions which shape their meanings, images of death in the later nineteenth and twentieth centuries can be seen as crucial in the construction of social identities. Here we examine the cultural practices of display to reveal their influence within the formation of both dominant ideologies of bodily control as well as the visual strategies through which these are subverted.

During the nineteenth century, post-mortem portraiture became widely available to middle and lower-middle classes so that images of deceased relatives were preserved in family albums and domestic display (Figure 7). As Townsend notes, there was a tendency to present the deceased in a lifelike manner so that the dead appeared, for instance, as though in sleep (1998: 131). In this respect such photographs drew on the conventions of earlier portrait painting. Indeed, Warner notes the continuities between 'media which transcribe bodies' – effigies, death masks and photography (Warner, 1995). Photographic images were used to record the end of life but also to overcome this end in that they provided the dead with a visible presence within domestic spaces. The physical features of particular family members were preserved, thereby providing a means by which a person was held within view and incorporated into the continuing life histories of relatives. Post-mortem photography therefore operated as a representation which provided a basis for the narrative reconstruction of the deceased's life.

The ritual surrounding death was also captured within these representations so that they record both the specificity of an event along with its social, personal and emotional impact. Ruby's study of nineteenth century American death photography reveals the visual documentation of funerary ritual (1995). Here the body of the deceased was photographed at the deathbed after it had been ritually prepared and dressed. Photographs of relatives at the deathbed, beside the coffin and at the graveside, record intense experiences of embodied grief in the form of images. As part of family collections the photograph stands as a material object to be viewed and contemplated within longer-term processes of grief and remembrance. Again, these visual images operate to inform the construction of life histories, emotional biographies and identities of kin groups. Of importance here is the way in which photographs form cultural representations which ensure that the dead remain socially active, that is, as a continued presence within the social and imaginative life of families (Gillis, 1997). This process of visual record-making and negotiation of memories associated with the dead runs counter to dominant perceptions of death as a marginalised aspect of social life.

While photographic images facilitated the development of rituals of death and remembrance within private spaces, further techniques of representation and display are central to the formation of attitudes towards the dead body in wider public domains. Although the private viewing of death in family photographs appears to be culturally acceptable, as are many public memorials to the war dead, public display can generate considerable controversy. The impact of visual representations of death centres on the perceived difference between the 'real' and the imaged body. While it might be argued that the production of visual images of the dead body acts as a distancing technique, providing a means to control and cope with an emotionally fraught life event, contemporary artists have begun to challenge the perceived boundaries between the 'real' and the imagined corpse.

Photography, with its claim to record what is 'real' has been used by artists to provide a public forum for the detailed examination of the physical aspects of death. For example the work of Sue Fox presents photographic images of corpses in the mortuary, a space which is usually secluded from public view. In an analysis of Fox's images, Townsend notes that:

> The mortuary is an environment where the body is reduced to an object of measurement by pathologists, where it becomes so much 'meat'....In this context the scientific, objective photograph would seem appropriate. But Fox's photographs subvert this objectification, in that through them she explores her own subjectivity, and in particular her 'fear of death'.
>
> (Townsend, 1988: 132)

Townsend goes on to claim that:

> Fox uses the corpse to signify ephemerality and loss of control. We like to think that we can extend ourselves infinitely, that

through science, self discipline or faith we can perfect and manage our bodies so that they will never die.

(ibid.: 132)

Fox's work is challenging and disturbing in that it presents visual evidence of the limits of the body, but at the same time it recovers the dead body as a site of public contemplation breaching the seclusion of the mortuary and therefore disrupting the authority of a specialised professional space. Through this work the corpse is made available for interpretation beyond the confines of expert control, a strategy which has been reinforced in recent exhibitions. For example, *In Visible Light. Photography and Classification in Art, Science and the Everyday*, held at the Museum of Modern Art, Oxford (1997), addressed issues in the relationships between photographs and dominant technological and scientific discourses. The exhibition of death photography here offered a commentary upon the interpretation of the dead body within clinical observation, scientific classification and media exploitation (Roberts, 1997: 33–38).

By relocating the corpse, through photographic images, within the art gallery, contemporary artists' strategies have aimed to confront the 'reality' of death within wider public domains. This has afforded them a role in rituals of death which sustain memories of the dead and therefore maintain the social presence of the deceased. Furthermore, Townsend argues that through death photography there is the possibility of 'identification between spectator and estranged subject, even a dying or deceased subject....we are interpellated into death through our relationship with others' (1998: 135). Such an identification does, however, depend upon the ways in which the corpse is represented. In this respect, we might note the work of photographer Rudolf Schafer whose photographs concentrate on the faces of women and men who 'died of natural causes', in an attempt to capture the 'peaceful' rest of ordinary death. His aim was to show 'what dead people look like' (1989: 193): a deliberate avoidance of sensational and exploitative imagery. In an interview which accompanied the publication of his images, he states:

[t]hese photographs may also seem strange because of the way I've presented them. A full-face portrait, perfectly natural in life, seems unnatural in death. These are ordinary poses. We are constantly bombarded with newspaper and television pictures

of catastrophes and wars – violent, extreme pictures – but we defuse one of the implications of these images – our own mortality – with the thought that nothing so extreme will ever happen to us. With these pictures you simply don't have that option.

(Schafer, 1989: 193)

Despite the intentions of contemporary artists in the contexts of exhibitions which seek to provide public access to the reality of death, issues of morality, legitimate ownership and control over the treatment of the corpse are vigorously contested. For instance, *The Art of Death* exhibition at the Victoria and Albert Museum planned for March 1991 was postponed. According to a newspaper report the museum authorities

decided that the Gulf War, and the prospect of numerous casualties, would be just the wrong moment to dwell on mortality. So the exhibition was put off until a time at which (it was anticipated) only the normal number of people would be dying.
(*The Independent* Magazine, 6 April 1991)

The reception of images of death is therefore, tied in significant ways to social and political contexts.

Furthermore, the display of the real corpse in museums, as opposed to effigies and images of the dead body has recently generated further public debate. *The Worlds of the Body* exhibition which opened in November 1997 at the State Museum for Labour and Technology in Mannheim, displayed 200 preserved human corpses (Figure 8). The exhibition was devised by Dr Gunter Van Hargens, whose stated aim was to reveal 'the "beauty" and the "vulnerability" of the human body' (*Time*, 15 December 1997). Corpses were displayed without skin or in horizontal or vertical sections, to reveal the complexity of anatomical structures. The curators claimed that the exhibition was 'educational' and 'aesthetic' and strong public interest was demonstrated by 125,000 visitors in five weeks. Diverse interpretations of the exhibition were reported: professional anatomists described it as 'perverse' and members of the Catholic and Evangelical churches in Mannheim claimed that it was 'not only grossly tasteless, but immoral, voyeuristic' (ibid.). At the heart of such debates lie questions regarding the fate of the corpse and the limits of public display. Exhibitions of this kind highlight uncertainties about the relationship between body and self and the extent to which any body can be viewed as an object.

Although the exhibition made direct and powerful claims to display the real or 'natural' body, in fact it provides us with another example of how cultural processes come into play. Through an advanced embalming process decay was arrested and the bodies were effectively frozen in time (an exercise in the display of power over natural processes of decomposition). The corpses were subjected to the scientific gaze, classified and enclosed within museum cabinets. While making claims to its educational potential, the exhibition effectively reinforced the authority of scientific and technological discourses. Control of the fate of the corpse acts as a sign of power. Responses to the display of the dead are again historically constituted.

While the display of the corpse might be read as a reinforcement of institutional authority, there are contexts in which the decaying body has been deployed within strategies of protest. Lincoln (1993) analyses the public display of exhumed bodies as a 'ritual of collective obscenity' in the years prior to the 1936 Spanish civil war. The opposition of the Left to the Church was expressed through the exhumation of bodies of priests, nuns and saints which were then displayed at altars. The ritual desecration of churches formed a violent resistance to ecclesiastical control. Lincoln draws out the social and symbolic significance of these spectacles in terms of the political construction of social groups. He interprets this ritual use of the dead and decaying bodies as an attempt to constitute a different social identity in opposition to the existing social order. This was achieved symbolically through the defilement of sacred space. Lincoln notes that, in an attempt to expose what they saw as the corruption of the Church, the protesters used a form of symbolic discourse rich in connotations of decay.

> The category of corruption is of considerable interest in the present context because like its near-synonyms rottenness and decadence, corruption is most concretely and emphatically manifest in the state of bodily decomposition. The most disquieting of all natural processes, bodily corruption comes inevitably with the passage of time as dead flesh putrefies and decays.
>
> (Lincoln, 1993: 125)

For the Church, physical decomposition signified sin and moral downfall. To bring decomposing corpses to the church altars operated on a symbolic level to reveal the profanity of a sacred institution. There were, of course, counter-interpretations of the ritual desecration of churches which represented the protests as instances of 'inhumanity', 'barbarity' and 'bestiality' (ibid.: 107). In this historical context, the corpse was imbued with potent political meanings and formed a significant symbolic resource through which conflicting political agendas were played out.

One further form of visual representation which exercises a powerful influence upon perceptions of the dead and dying body in contemporary society is the contemporary horror film. Here, the dying and dead body forms a resource for fantasies in which extreme violence is inflicted. For example, the dismemberment, radical metamorphosis and destruction of the body is repeatedly revealed. Drawing upon Kristeva's theory of abjection, Creed (1995) discusses the ways in which the destruction of the body in horror films operates on a symbolic level to destroy all cultural values. Kristeva defines the corpse as 'the utmost of abjection' and elaborates further: 'It is thus not lack of cleanliness or health that causes abjection but what disturbs identity, system, order. What does not respect borders, positions, roles. The in-between, the ambiguous, the composite' (1982: 4). The visual representation of the corpse in films then constitutes a threat to social boundaries and systems of exclusion which seek to control disorderly bodies. In Creed's discussion of the cinema of horror she argues that the horror film's obsession with the materiality of the body is linked to 'an obsession with the nature of the self' (Creed, 1995: 143). Creed argues that horror appears to attack the notion of the unified rational self in that spectators are invited to view the destruction of the body as if it were their own. It is here that images of the dead body become potentially subversive; the corpse becomes the vehicle through which the breaking of taboos and societal constraints is explored.

On the other hand, horror films function to reaffirm viewers' perception of their own bodies as 'clean' and 'whole'. Given that horror films ultimately fail to sustain the identification of the viewer, in that they are recognised as fictions, one of their ideological agendas is to mark the difference between the 'pure' body and its 'abject other'. This effectively provides for the spectator a 'reaffirmation of a comforting but illusory sense of a unified, coherent, authentic body and self' (Creed, 1995: 156–157).

On balance, the dynamics between the film's representation of the corpse and its reception by viewers tends to reproduce dominant conceptions of the self in relation to a bounded, clean body.

Conclusions

Via this examination of European visual cultures of death, a range of issues have been introduced. Representations of the dead and dying body have been shown to impinge directly upon embodied experience. However, the nature of visual representation is historically and culturally variable and complex systems of reference and allusion are deployed through images of the dead and dying body. Yet analysis of the ways in which images operate over time reveals the persistent production of visual imagery around the dead body. These images refer to one another in that conventions are lifted from one form of representation to be deployed in another, for example, the convention of death as mirror. Such images might reinforce or work against one another. Similarly, images of the body in crisis are taken up and deployed within wider discourses: moralising, spiritual, political, and scientific. Relationships between representation and spectator are shaped by these wider discourses as images are embedded in particular social and cultural contexts and meanings are invoked in different ways. With regard to representations of death, Bronfen and Goodwin raise key questions:

> Many of the cultural systems concerned with death are in fact constructed to give a voice to the silenced dead. The question might be asked, Who or what represents the corpse?[...]On the one hand, it can mean, How do we represent the point at which a body becomes a corpse? What is the truth-value of the technological response(s) to this question? And even here we might well ask who 'we' are who is doing the representing, to what audience, for what purpose. How is the corpse represented differently for the purposes of law, of mourning, of the news media, of aestheticization in a symbol?
>
> (Bronfen and Goodwin, 1993: 6)

In foregrounding such questions they also emphasise the cultural politics which often underpin visual images. 'Representations of death necessarily engage questions of power: its locus, its authenticity, its sources and how it is passed on. The very mobility and instability of power help undermine the simplistic binaries of life and death' (ibid.: 4–5).

As we have suggested, images of the dying and dead body have been used, depending on historical context, to either reinforce a sense of social order or as a means to instigate social disorder. The metaphorical potential of the body and, in particular the damaged or fragmented body, has been exploited in a variety of ways through the production and dissemination of visual representations. These images have been used to articulate social and cultural connections which reinforce a sense of continuity of self within wider social and moral orders. On the other hand, they have also been used to articulate disconnection and political opposition to particular regimes and institutions. Further, they have been mobilised in attempts to reinforce structures of authority in that dominant discourses make claims on the body in death as territory to be controlled. While we might observe this strategy in the maintenance of power relations, images of the body in death have also been used to dismantle or critique hierarchies of power. We are therefore faced with a profusion of visual images and material objects relating to the dead and dying body. These images set up particular sets of relationships between the represented body and the real body – so that what is understood by the 'reality' of death is alluded to in different ways. In other words these images claim different degrees of transparency. They therefore set up different relationships between the image and the viewer shaping social practice and embodiment in a variety of ways. Attention has to be paid to the ways in which representations work – how they accrue contextual meanings and how codes and conventions develop over time, how they are deployed in strategies of control and subversion and how they impinge on the formation of self and social identity.

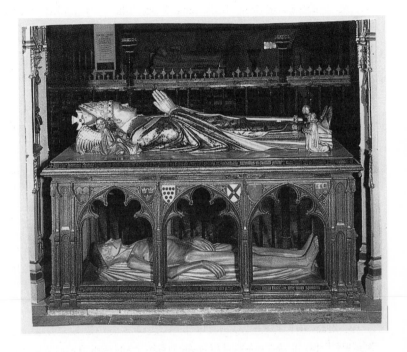

Figure 1   The tomb of Archbishop Henry Chichele (c. 1425),
Canterbury Cathedral.

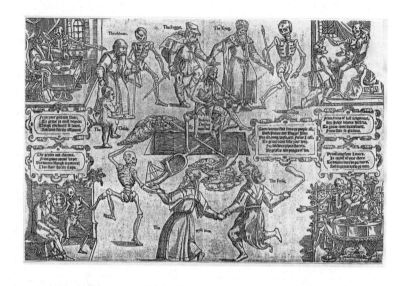

Figure 2 'The daunce and song of death' (1569). Collection of ballads in the British Library, reprinted by Joseph Lilley, 1867.

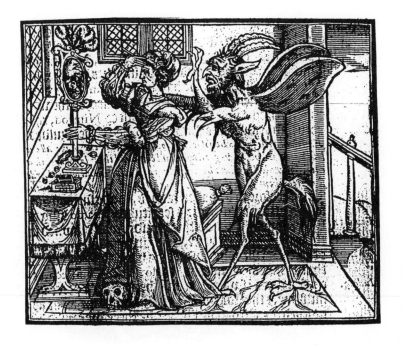

Figure 3   'The Description of Pride' (1569).

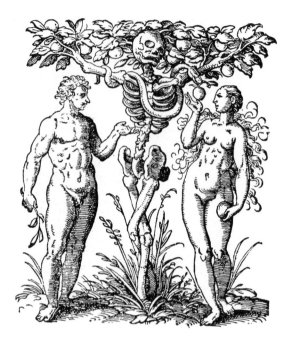

Figure 4 'The Tree of Knowledge and Death' (1587).

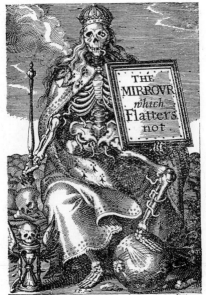

O that they were Wise, that they vnderſtood This, that they would Conſider their latter End ! Deut: 32 29

Figure 5   'The Mirror which Flatters Not' (1639).

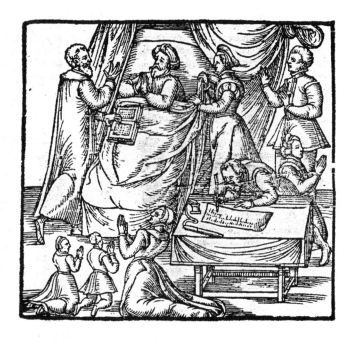

Figure 6 Deathbed scene from 'The crie of the poore for the death of the Right Honourable Earle of Huntingdon' (1596).

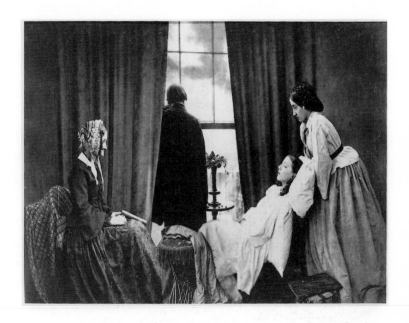

Figure 7 'Fading Away', Henry Peach Robinson (1858). Albumen print. Ruby
(1995) notes the continuities between postmortem photography
and representations of grief in nineteenth century romantic painting
as well as pictorialist photographs, for example Robinson's
composite photograph.

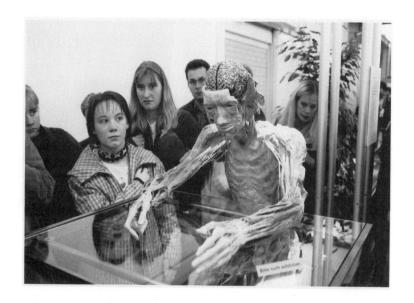

Figure 8   Photograph of an exhibit at 'The Worlds of the Body' Exhibition,
State Museum for Technology and Labour, Mannheim, Germany
(1997).

Chapter 3

Bodies without selves

Images of embodied human life in its final stages often include the housebound widow, at risk of dying alone and undiscovered; the greying bodies which line the lounges of residential homes; and the eerie moans of the frail elderly who clog hospital beds. Represented in this way, such individuals come to be constructed as 'other'. They are seen to have lost their place in society and now find themselves accommodated among individuals who have never had one – for example, people who have had long institutional lives as a result of physical and mental disability. The concept of 'social death', previously used to describe the breakdown of social interaction between dying patients and their families (Glaser and Strauss, 1965, 1968; Sudnow, 1967), has now been extended to incorporate such individuals. Mulkay describes the socially dead as those who have 'ceased to exist as an active agent in the ongoing social world of some other party' (1993: 33).

This chapter takes up the theoretical implications of the Foucauldian argument that the human body comes to be produced within a range of discourses and that, in their plurality, such discourses produce a layered multiplicity of body readings. According to this view, the old, grey body lying undiscovered in the council flat, can be an initiation for a new police constable or trainee funeral director, a stimulus for depression among older neighbours, a source of shame for social workers and a reproach for estranged family members. Even in less extreme circumstances, older bodies can be understood as a locus for tension between discourses – for example, generalised stereotypes of 'the elderly' as opposed to personalised, historicised family identities. It has been argued that these discourses produce different kinds of body, self-identity and phenomenological experiences of self. This chapter makes Foucault's conception of 'discourse' its starting point but raises critical questions about the relationship between cultural representations and social practices. In pursuing this theoretical agenda, we ask how the old body which is understood as 'living' comes to be transformed into the old body which is understood as 'corpse'. What emerges is a fluidity of body readings, produced through both discourse and practice, an effect of dominant systems of power as well as evidence of their instability in the face of resistance.

Critiques of a Foucauldian view suggest that under the weight of external social influences, or discourses, the material and phenomenological body begins to disappear. Shilling, for example, argues that this form of social constructionism takes no account of the biological aspects of embodiment, nor does it represent the body as both a resource for and a constraint upon individual agency (1993). The ageing, dying and dead body provides a particularly salient focus when examining the tension between these views in that its materiality is not just in evidence, but problematically so. Moreover, there are questions as to the degree to which older adults are able to resist or participate in externally imposed discourses and social practices such as medicalisation or welfarism. The focus of this chapter is therefore the old body as a site of tension within which competing representations and practices seek to claim ascendancy. Of particular interest is the theoretical puzzle regarding the possibility of a mismatch between 'self' as somatised at the body's surface and 'self' as an internally experienced subjectivity. How can we understand the experience of feeling many years younger than others assume us to be? While the concept of social death highlights an externally imposed exclusion, it does not necessarily illuminate the experience itself, nor the ways in which it may be resisted. Of core interest, therefore, is the tension between the production of self via its exterior bodily form and the experience of the self via embodiment.

This chapter asks about the social identities of those who discover themselves in a marginal social position as a result of changes to their bodies which are associated with the approach of death. It develops this volume's theoretical agenda by asking how we might make sense of the self-diminishment which appears to take place among the socially 'dead', or at least 'dying'; those individuals thought to survive in bodily but not social form. If 'self' and 'body' are largely synonymous, as current theorists argue, then very old and deteriorating bodies will be unlikely sites of enselvement (Turner, 1998). Yet while the term 'social death' may usefully describe the severity of isolation experienced by marginal individuals, it does not tell us much about aspects of their existence which may be at odds with a deathly self-identity. The chapter therefore has two objectives. First, it provides an account of 'social death' not as an event or a state, but as a process of social positioning which is carried out largely by younger people in relation to elders. Second, while acknowledging those aspects of older adults' lives which constitute a form of social death, it also provides a more nuanced approach to the lives which they none the less lead. Recognising the multiplicity of discourses and practices through which old bodies are being produced, it asks about the social presence of older adults in a symbolic sense, that is, the meanings and effects of their presence. It also asks about their social being in phenomenological terms; and about the intentions and actions of older people which are often overlooked within conventional uses of the term 'agency'. In particular, the chapter argues that, as a result of the theoretical privileging of embodied social interaction as the core of social participation, those aspects of cognitive and imaginative social life which fall outside its spotlight are made marginal. Concepts of 'social interaction' and 'social death' are therefore interrogated in order to account for the embodied experience of dying.

Reading the 'finished' body

In Chapter 1 we discussed Shilling's view of the body as 'an entity which is in the process of becoming' (1993), that is as an unfinished product which is socially, as well as biologically, constituted. Further, if we follow Giddens (1991), we can recognise a distinctively Western 'finishing' of the body, the outcome of a reflexive process whereby the body is made to contribute to a consciously chosen social identity. These theoretical perspectives have been developed from work on the gendered, the sexual, the healthy, the deviant and the consuming body. They are the yet-to-be finished bodies which reveal Western society's members at work on their individual projects. When it comes to the old or dying body there seems less to say. The production of chosen self-identities appears to flourish only in younger adulthood since the body, as a material resource, can be made to yield a desired self for a limited period only. None the less, if we return to Shilling's original proposal – that it is our engagement within social life which 'finishes' the body – then it is insufficient merely to cite the forms of body-identity work which enhance or sustain favoured social identities. By implication, those with old bodies have either given up the struggle or carry out their projects with markedly less success. Yet if theorists of embodiment limit the scope of bodies selected for discussion, they are working from a partial picture. As will be argued, it is a picture which reinforces existing relations of power and inequality and moreover leaves us with an under-theorised account of later life embodiment. Theorists such as Bryan Turner (1984) have described the body as the product of discourse, an entity which comes into being through a micro-politics of power. When bodies are old and frail, it is easy to see how in becoming subject to discourses surrounding a concept such as 'social death', the subjectivities of women and men themselves begin to lose substance.

Studies have revealed that, even at birth (as demonstrated in substantially different birth weights) social factors have an effect on the body (Wilkinson, 1996). In later life an entire social history can be read off the old body – in the lines of the face; in scarring from childbirth, accidents and surgery; and in the way clothing is worn and everyday tasks are performed. However, the workings of the social and cultural environment upon the body are only part of the story of later life. In reading the old body, one is not reading an inactive body – even though its 'activities' may be invisible to those attuned to the vigorous actions of earlier life. Instead, the earlier imperative to construct a high status, youthful and attractive body can be superseded by more important concerns such as the management of losses – short-term memory, good eyesight, the limb's flexibility or the fingers dexterity. Matthews (1979) provided an early account of these practices in her work on old women and identity maintenance where she identified the strategies through which women succeeded in repairing age-based damage to their personae. Discussing Giddens' analysis, Shilling describes dying as the failure of the body project, the point 'where human control ends in a world which is orientated to the successful achievement of control' (1993: 184). As this chapter will show, this view provides only limited insight into the embodied experiences of older, and indeed, dying individuals. More than any other, the old body is socially constituted. Not only does it carry a layering, indeed sedimentation, of social thought and action within its physical frame, but in its demands upon the individual, it is a project requiring sometimes continuous application.

Here we begin to grapple with tensions which are core to this chapter and focus particularly upon the multiplicity of readings to which the old body may be subject. What we argue is that issues of power become ever more central as the body ages. Featherstone and Hepworth (1991) in their concept of a 'mask of ageing', highlight the privileging of the outer body as the source of a negative self-identity. As a result, older people experience a mis-reading of their bodies in that a bent and wrinkled exterior conceals the youthful self which they may themselves experience, subjectively. This is exemplified in J.B. Priestley's sense of shock at his mirror image, one which in no sense reflects his inner self-experience (Featherstone and Hepworth, 1991: 379). On the one hand, stereotypical and stigmatising images of older people proliferate within an ageist, youth-oriented society. These suggest the occurrence of a series of pre-mortal death states. On the other hand, testimonies to an internally generated sense of self belie the negativity of such appearances. What we seem to have, therefore, is a problematic juxtaposition of theories of old age. In the former, marginalised older people undergo a 'social death' which denies the possibility of any form of social participation; in the latter, the metaphor of a 'mask of ageing' highlights older people's subjective sense of self which remains vividly, albeit painfully, alive.

In arguing that embodiment in later life is like wearing a mask, Featherstone and Hepworth highlight the failure of the body's competencies which militate against effective participation in social life. Loss of facial muscle tone, hearing and eyesight undermine the sense of timing necessary for effective conversation (1991: 376). Privileged here is a set of biological changes which, in contemporary Western society, gradually inhibit social participation. However, sources such as the work of poet and playwright, Tony Harrison (1993), are a reminder that many of the conditions of old age – for example, Alzheimer's disease – are problematic, at least in part, as a result of the privileging of rational verbal interaction in today's society. His work shows that while other personal attributes such as a sense of rhythm and a feeling for touch and music carry less weight in terms of the maintenance of social identity, these are faculties which may well endure in the person with Alzheimer's disease, someone often positioned as socially dead and grieved for long in advance of their bodily death.

The separation of physical body and self-identity arguably characterises the experience of many older people. Indeed, in the case of monarchs and celebrities this separation is made public and visible. As detailed in Chapter 2, the funerary art of late medieval England juxtaposed representations of the elite dead in full possession of their social faculties with images of the decaying corpse (Llewellyn, 1991). With a focus on living monarchs, Barthes identifies press revelations of the 'human' face of royalty as a way of underscoring their aristocratic status:

> To flaunt the fact that kings are capable of prosaic actions is to recognize that this status is no more natural to them than angelism to common mortals, it is to acknowledge that the king is still king by divine right.
>
> (1973: 32–33)

However, when the individual is a more ordinary mortal the identity which they value is seen to be locked within them, rather than raised above them on the open surface of a tomb or spread across the front page of a newspaper. What takes precedence is a deteriorating physical body and an associated set of readings which is at odds with their subjective sense of self. This raises the question of whether the term 'socially dead' is an appropriate description of those whose appearances belie their subjective experience, whose bodily control is minimal or absent, whose social interactions are vastly different from those expected among younger adults. We suggest that 'social death' should not be seen as a state or an event, but perhaps more accurately a social process through which people who are socially disadvantaged become marginalised. Crucially, it is their bodies which provide the evidence of their less than full social identity. Freund has argued that the experience and appearance of the body can provide 'manifestations' and 'prototypes' of ideas about how the body should look and behave which in turn feed back into structures of power and inequality (cited in Shilling, 1993: 117). Thus, in a society where slender, mobile, smooth-skinned bodies are a social and economic asset, the sight of individuals who are bent and slow-moving with slack, wrinkled skin shores up a generalised stereotype that older people are no longer fully alive in a social sense, that they make poor companions, demanding family members and unreliable work mates. These assumptions then feed in to the positioning of older people, both structurally and in everyday encounters.

Social death is therefore an imposed condition. It may be imposed to the extent that the individual experiences a strong sense of
alienation or marginalisation. Or it may be felt but resisted by
individuals for whom embodied life as a social being remains vital if
demanding. The metaphor of a mask to connote the ageing body
does, however, testify strongly to the experience of a tension
between the self and the body at the point at which the body is no
longer experienced as an authentic representation of the self. Turner
brings a temporal perspective to bear when he highlights the
importance of embodied memory as an aspect of growing older. The
passage of time, he suggests, can be experientially measured in the
deteriorating body, which itself becomes 'a walking memory' (1995:
250). The world of consciousness in later life is therefore, in
Turner's words, a nostalgic world filled with 'the yearning for a
particular body in its youthful habitus' (ibid.: 251). The reflexivity
which characterises human subjectivity would therefore seem to
permit the existence of a plurality of bodies, lived, remembered and
imposed. That they may at times be in tension with one another is
manifested most graphically in responses to the death of key public
figures. As already noted, the tenuousness of elite social power can
be overcome by making the social body *atemporal* in preserved
images of the live body in fitness and health – in tombs and
paintings of monarchs, in obituary photographs of great women and
men and in media re-runs of the film stars, celebrities and European
royalty who are its objects. And in silent obscurity we find the
abject body, once depicted in slow decay on the underside of tombs
(Kristeva, 1982). In the example of Diana, Princess of Wales, her
invisible corpse was everywhere brought to mind, a powerful absent
presence. It was there in the sustained exposure of close-up media
images of its coffin, in graphic accounts of its medical treatment
prior to death and in the titillating news of censored photographs of
her dying body. Once her decaying corpse was secured below
ground on a private, uninhabited island, her social self, or 'image',
was free to continue its existence, its value if anything augmented
by the off-stage presence of its deteriorating shadow self.

Through the examples which follow we examine the theoretical
propositions discussed above. In every case a multiplicity of voices
and practices make themselves heard, felt and at times resisted. By
examining specific examples, this chapter will attend to those
neglected aspects of the life of old bodies: their symbolic potency;
their role as vehicles for embodied experience; and their agency.

From social theories of the body we take the notion of the body as project and argue that current work neglects those projects which do not appear to yield a satisfactory self-identity. Two key projects which older people in contemporary Western society engage with in relation to their bodies are the management of health and the management of approaching death and it is to examples relating to both these projects that we now turn.

'Health' as project in later life

The imperative for self-care brought in by the new public health has, on some level, proved irresistible for people of all ages (Lupton, 1996). Good health is unanimously highlighted by body-as-project theorists as the holy grail of embodied self-realisation (see, for example, Featherstone, 1991: 183). Over time, however, its meanings vary. For example, it can range from 'health' as a prerequisite for an attractive appearance – 'looking good, feeling great' – through to more functional notions of fitness and well-being (Coward, 1984). However, in later life, when 'health' is no longer a given, it can begin to constitute a different kind of project (Conway and Hockey, 1998). Thus research shows older people asserting their 'good health' (Sidell, 1995), if only as a claim made in the face of expectations that being old and being ill are one and the same thing; they therefore declare their unusual luck, sound self-care or a good genetic inheritance. In that illness and old age are often elided and the good health of old bodies cannot be assumed, it represents an area of potential body 'work' for many older adults.

What is particularly crucial here is that, despite a proliferation of sickness-based identities – AIDS victim; junkie; battered wife; schizophrenic, the social identity of older adults in fact remains ambiguous with regard to health. Paradoxically, it is the centrality of the concept of 'sickness' to prevailing notions of old age that renders it an implicit, taken-for-granted aspect of what has become a highly medicalised period of the life course (Armstrong, 1981). What predominates in later life identities is AGE, as evidenced in titles such as senior citizen, old age pensioner, or older adult; and in age-specific adjectives such as 'active', 'spry', 'sprightly', or 'game'. These adjectives, in highlighting the vigour of a particular older adult, silently connote their less lively peers. We can compare the case of younger adults, where illness is thought of as a departure from normality. It is this which is so readily recognised in Talcott Parsons' model of the 'sick role' – a strictly delimited time of legitimated deviance (1951).

Having some kind of chronic sickness, disability or degeneration is therefore seen as an unsurprising aspect of later life. Although the 'socially dead' may experience their bodies as intensely if problematically alive, these same bodies are often imagined as silent and passive by younger adults. In reality, pain may be inescapable, limits on mobility and on the senses may make older people acutely aware of their embodiment; loss of control – in falling, in incontinence, in slurred speech, in drooling – renders the body visible and gives it a powerful social presence. As Leder notes, pain disrupts our normal experience of 'bodily disappearance', making the body central to our consciousness in an alien and dysfunctional manner (Leder, cited in Williams and Bendelow, 1998). The old body can therefore be experienced as an object of consuming interest for the individual.

At the beginning of this chapter it was argued that much of the current work on the body neglects the older body and in so doing fails to provide an account of its symbolic power, its phenomenology, and its agency. To take up the first of these areas, we turn to the work of anthropologist, Mary Douglas, to consider its symbolic or meaning-making power (1966). Important here is the old body's domain of influence, its power as a symbol or representation. We need to ask how this power is felt and deployed within society. By limiting the vision of social engagement simply to active, face-to-face interaction, little can be said about the place of the body in shaping and influencing the sphere of thought and feeling, the habitus within which all bodies are 'finished'.

For Mary Douglas, however, the body is an intimate material resource within and through which the social body can be symbolised. Shilling argues that her work tends to collapse the social and physical body in such a way that the phenomenology of the individual body is reduced to 'the positions and categories made available by the social body' (1993: 73). None the less, by focusing on specific examples of the old body's symbolising potential, it remains possible to access its phenomenological counterpart. Douglas's work on the body as a classificatory system is valuable in alerting us to the importance of the body as a (re)source for meaning-making and therefore as an important aspect of the ways in which the individual participates in society.

As argued above, issues of power lie at the heart of the way in which the older body is positioned, both socially and culturally. Not only are we dealing with the manner in which old bodies figure within younger adults' symbolic systems as a representation of, for example, stupidity, self-neglect or human mortality – but also with the ways older people themselves may subvert or supplant such systems with sets of meanings of their own.

We have suggested that old age and illness are often elided within the discourses of younger adults, even though older adults may assert a state of 'good health' (Sidell, 1995). This point can be taken further. Illness in old age is often naturalised. That is to say, the illnesses of older adults are represented as the body's natural decline, and indeed, the old body and the natural world are often collapsed through sets of mutually reflecting metaphors which valorise the gentle decline of the ageing 'other'. The old body is therefore 'in the autumn of its days', a season which has been romanticised in poetic language such as Keat's 'season of mists and mellow fruitfulness' where ripeness and maturity elegantly mask deterioration and decay. Not only the annual cycle of the seasons but also the daily cycle of morning and evening are drawn upon (Hockey and James, 1993). For example, in Scotland, residential homes for older adults are known as 'Eventide Homes'. Sutcliffe, the photographer, entitled his image of a young child nestled in an old man's arms, 'Morning and Evening'. Diurnal and annual temporal rhythms are thereby connoted. Being cyclical they do not suggest termination but rather acceptable change. In this way the bodily deterioration which is implicitly taken-for-granted as an aspect of later life is naturalised and indeed romanticised. Like the setting sun or the falling leaf, the body gently declines. Hence the perennial resonance of Tennyson's 'Choric Song of the Lotus-Eaters'. Here the approach of death is represented through metaphors of the natural world which render it plausibly desirable to the drugged consciousnesses of the lotus-eaters:

> Why should we only toil,
> the roof and crown of things...
> the full-juiced apple, waxing over-mellow,
> drops in a silent autumn night.
> All its allotted length of days, the flower ripens in its place,
> ripens and fades and falls, and hath no toil,

fast-rooted in the fruitful soil.
                    (Williams and Vallins, 1931: 23)

These representations of the old body as an aspect of a self-renewing cycle of nature, a form of embodiment within which illness leads only to a new turn of the wheel, can be set alongside a reading of the old body as childlike (Hockey and James, 1993). Again, the power of its enfeeblement is defused, this time through an implicit association with contemporary Western childhood conceived of as a period of change and growth characterised by clumsiness and lack of control – but in a temporary sense only.

In both these examples we find the old body invested with symbolic meanings which play an important part in the younger adult's contemplation of their own future. An awareness of impending illness or disability, to be followed by personal annihilation, is deflected and in its place the old body is made to connote two desirable realms – the natural world and the time of childhood.

Older people themselves, however, retain the possibility of subverting or supplanting this set of symbols. Anthropological field research carried out within a local authority residential home for older adults in the North East of England provides insights into the symbolising power of the body (Hockey, 1990). These data show that the imposition of a childlike nature, however comforting for younger adults, is costly for adults who have previously grown out of their childish ways. However, they can, and do, turn it to their advantage, for example in claiming licence for behaviours such as sticking out the tongue to members of staff, demanding to be wheeled around in a chair rather than having to walk, fussing over food in a way which would cause embarrassment in earlier life, telling tales on one another to the Officer in Charge and refusing to comply with staff's requests.

As well as subverting the ways in which particular readings of the old body are imposed upon them, older adults can supplant such meanings. For example, they made references to themselves as rubbish which could appropriately be placed in the black bin liners which staff used to gather sweepings from the floor, so connoting industrial waste rather than organic regeneration. More positively, embodied skills and practices from earlier life were reinstated in new forms. Thus a resident who had been a music teacher conducted the 'choir' of inarticulate and physically disabled residents; a middle-class woman 'visited' sick residents and sought to place staff in the role of lady's maids who were to tend her clothing; former Free Church committee members organised the residents' committee.

While many of these older adults had undergone some form of social death in being excluded from their former social roles, many of them now lacking an active family context, this term fails to account for the embodied selves which are evidenced in this material. Phenomenologically, it is clear that these individuals had a strong sense of their own subjectivity. They reflected upon their position in a way which is strikingly at odds with that of younger people. Rather than feeling excluded from the living, they noted the strangeness of remaining alive when 'most of my friends are dead'; 'all my generation has gone now, only the dregs are left' (Hockey, 1990: 109–110). When it came to their embodied experience they took questions of health every bit as seriously as younger adults, however, and in no sense saw themselves gently falling to the ground like ripened fruit. Thus they spoke of the corridors they had to 'walk up and down'; 'it does us good'. They massaged their bodies, they decided whether or not they should get up in the morning, often in tension with staff's wishes; they regarded their food with suspicion, being unwilling to eat 'scrapings'; they refused their pills if these caused unwanted side-effects, having a model of health which admitted to the possibility of death but warded off unnecessary suffering; they claimed their baths when they wanted them and they insisted on control of their hairstyles (ibid.).

In all this we have clear evidence of older people's agency. Again, it operated in sometimes contradictory modes, tending at times to be powerful in ways which were also costly. Thus older people would flaunt the breaching of their bodies boundaries in ways which powerfully subverted the highly bounded nature of residential life; they might defecate in sinks and corridors, refuse to walk to toilets in a bid for a wheelchair, roam the corridors at night or 'escape' the home. Similarly they would feign deafness or, if already deaf, raise their voices repeatedly. Ultimately powerful by virtue of their age and closeness to death, they were intractable and indeed ungovernable. For every resident who fell in the corridor, four staff were needed to haul them onto their feet; for every resident who refused to get out of bed, two or more were needed to persuade them otherwise, the time taken being ill-afforded within a hard-pressed institution. For every resident who allowed urine, faeces, saliva or mucus to escape their bodies, there was a uniform to be washed, a staff member who, privately, felt sullied and, in the case of faeces, who earned 30p extra pay as an acknowledgement of the 'contagion' they had been subjected to.

This is an example of what Victor Turner calls the 'power of the weak' (1974). The resource of a deteriorating body which could be subversively deployed. Data also revealed other forms of agency which sustained the social identity of the individuals concerned. Thus residents would 'care' for one another, selecting friends who were manageably less competent than themselves and avoiding those who were beyond them in terms of confusion or incontinence. In one case two women married their remaining faculties in such a way that they became a composite embodied person, the one having good eyesight, and the other a strong set of legs (Hockey, 1990).

The near departed

In early or mid-life, the occurrence of death is even more aberrant than illness. The adjectives used to describe the deaths of children or younger adults – 'untimely', 'tragic' or 'wasteful' – are highly age-specific and would sit uneasily in the context of an older person's death. However, despite the deferral of death to later life, older adults may not be explicitly categorised as 'dying' – merely as 'old'. While some of them may depend upon the care of others, few are likely to be receiving 'terminal' or 'palliative' care (Komaromy and Hockey, in press). Yet the age-based life course category to which they belong is singled out as the one which by definition lies in close temporal proximity to death. In addition to an assumed state of poor health, therefore, those with old bodies are also implicitly assumed to be faced with the proximity of death. Indeed, so 'natural' is death in later life that older people's fear of their own death, and their grief at the loss of their contemporaries, often remains invisible (Hockey, 1990; Howarth 1998).

If the imminent demise of the near departed is constructed as unremarkable, this is not to say that the nature of their fate is insignificant. Although uneventful when seen from the perspective of younger people, we still need to ask how society in general imagines the events which overtake older people. What is thought to happen to their bodies and what is envisaged for them as individuals? Here we argue that the way in which concepts such as 'life' and 'death', and their relationship with one another, are understood is important as an aspect of what is meant by later life. As indicated earlier, this volume sets out to question the conceptualisation of life and death as a binary opposition with life taking the hierarchically superior position in relation to death (Grosz, 1989). Here we argue that this dichotomy produces a stigmatising view of older people as fast approaching a kind of crunch point at which positively perceived life is utterly transformed into negatively perceived death. It is the increasingly differentiated nature of what are constructed as two readily juxtaposed categories which is important here. While the goal of life's earlier body projects, the maintenance of a fit and attractive body, deflects awareness of mortality, the projects of later life are undertaken very much with mortality in mind; in the form of making wills, resolving troubled social relationships and disposing of items not intended for a public gaze. Even though Bauman notes that 'we do not hear of people dying of mortality' (1992: 138), and Prior has documented the increasing categorisation of death as the product of specific cases of organ failure (1989), human mortality and the concept of 'natural' death cannot be fully repressed. This is evidenced in the taken-for-granted proliferation of female corpses in Western art and literature. Bronfen argues that in a patriarchal society the young woman's body, in its 'otherness', provides a localised site within which the irrepressible universality of human mortality can safely be contemplated. Old bodies, arguably, are a more ambiguous local site in being both profoundly 'other', yet simultaneously offering a representation of all our future selves. The deferral of death to old age is therefore an acknowledgement of our two-faced encounter with death – as beings who know of, yet cannot imagine their own finitude. In being confined to its place among older people, the rampant epidemic of death is made more or less acceptable.

This set of assumptions, we argue, provides the complex cultural and social context within which old bodies are read. About to become corpses, these bodies testify to the inevitable extinction of the self which they are seen to represent. As Turner (1995) argues, in Western societies the body's surface has become an indicator of the individual's moral condition. Inherited from nineteenth century scientific discourses of madness, criminality and sexuality, contemporary forms of regulatory knowledge such as child development schedules, sex manuals and fitness regimes blur into a more generalised notion that the inner self can be accessed via the body's external appearance. In the case of the lined and bent body we find a representation of an age-based social identity which implies a proximity to the negatively perceived half of the life:death binary. It is therefore unsurprising that this 'deathly' appearance is readily assumed to encompass a socially dead self.

The data which showed that older people were engaged in the 'project' of health also suggest that they may be simultaneously drawn into projects concerned with death (Hockey, 1990). Here the power of younger adult discourses is in evidence, older adults being subject to forms of surveillance, by both staff and other residents, which resulted in their categorisation as either 'fit' or 'frail' residents. By implication, those who were 'fit' were those who remained in many respects socially alive. Staff said that they had come into care in order to 'make a new home for themselves' and indeed they found roles which corresponded to their earlier engagement with family, church, local community and place of work. The 'frail', however, were variously constructed as 'socially dead'. Other residents 'disinherited' them. One emaciated, confused resident, for example, was shunned by others who would describe her as 'not one of mine'. Such residents were referred to by care staff as 'vegetables', 'dying ducks' and 'little dolls' who were 'away with the show folks'. Their marginal status was highlighted in the commonly used phrase, 'on her way out', a notion of movement which reflected both the exit of the self from the body as well as the body's passage from sick bay to morgue to crematorium.

The distinction between 'fit' and 'frail' was crucial within the residential home, an institutionalised space located within a society where life and death are made to stand in a dichotomous relationship to one another. It represented a strategy whereby the implicitly death-like status of the 'old' could be managed, the ever-present nature of human mortality thereby continuing to be deferred – for just a little longer. However, it constituted a social strategy which was continuously confounded by the old body's materiality. Residents categorised as 'vegetables' might revive. They surfaced from sick bay and took their place at dining tables where they ate heartily. 'Little dolls' danced with the Friends of the Home. And upstairs, the 'fit' would die without warning, their bodies seated in a wheelchair, being brought down in the home's small lift. This act disturbed staff in that it confounded the separation of 'life' and 'death' via the ambiguous image of the seated corpse.

Residents' old bodies not only stood for a condition of near departure; they were also a resource which older individuals could mobilise in resistance to the notion of social death. For example, residents would 'play' dead, crossing their arms corpse-like on their chests when staff brought in the early morning cup of tea. They would take off jewellery conspicuously, reminding staff that the body they were handling would soon be in the hands of funeral directors – and residents were safeguarding those body 'appendages' which they knew were valuable. Expected to be calmly acquiescent in the face of death, those residents who made their fear of imminent death known to staff were told that such fears were groundless. Jokes and deflections were commonplace but resisted by residents who frequently flung a reference to their imminent departure in the direction of a care assistant who was about to set off on another task.

So potent are the older bodies described here, and so 'vital' the interactions that surround them, that we are again forced to reconsider the theoretical debates raised at the outset of this chapter and ask about the extent to which the social self can be detached from the body in the way that Mulkay suggests (1993). In her work on the destruction of the self as a result of the radical breakdown of the body's surfaces during terminal illness, Lawton argues strongly for the possibility of a psychic death which pre-dates bodily death (1998). In circumstances of overwhelming helplessness and despair the self ceases to be. All that remains is an 'empty' body. This position forces us to re-think Featherstone and Hepworth's argument for a split between an external mask and a concealed, youthful inner self (1991). As a young female researcher, Barbara Myerhoff experimented with the experience of an old body through deliberate use of make-up, ear plugs, heavy shoes and thick glasses when going out in public (1978). This gave her insight into the way social interaction between younger and older adults results in the imposition of a 'mask' behind which an older person's younger self, in a phenomenological sense, comes to be concealed. Was Myerhoff somehow less socially alive when 'masked'? If social interaction is privileged in definitions of social identity, then her diminished interactional competencies as an 'old' woman constitute social death, at least in a minor form. However, if the retention of personal choice as to how the external body is presented negates the categorisation, 'socially dead', then by implication the existence of some kind of separate subjectivity is an important qualifier in the use of this term.

It is this inner world of individual subjectivities which has for long been foresworn by social scientists. In his work on post divorce narratives, Simpson (1998) highlights the persistent social presence of individuals who are absent from their former nuclear families, showing how the personal accounts of remaining family members contain 'traces of other people occupying other positions'. He argues that social relationships exist in the absence of face-to-face interaction, that we need to take account of the worlds of consciousness which exist alongside the worlds of action. Too often left outside the scope of the social sciences, with their emphasis on observable outer behaviours, the inner world of imagination and intentionality demands our attention (Cohen and Rapport, 1995). These authors warn against:

> the fundamental impropriety and inadequacy of taking consciousness for granted, and treating it as merely derivable from public manifestations of culture and behaviour: that is, of neglecting the contact zone, on the mistaken grounds that there is only one realm.
>
> (1995: 10)

Here we argue that it is the shadow side of observable reality which needs to be examined in order to make sense of the relationship between body and social identity among people who are old, dying or dead.

Conclusion

Focusing on the old body, this chapter has explored the question of social identity when the body has become extremely frail and/or brain function has diminished. It has asked how the metaphor of death – as in the notion of 'social death' – acquires the rhetorical power to define the social position of many older adults. It also questioned the assumed temporal sequence of social death followed by physical death. Later chapters will show how this temporal sequencing remains problematic, even for those whose bodies are more unequivocally characterised as 'dying'.

Through accounts of the embodied social lives of older people, we suggest that the concept of social death misleadingly prioritises agency, interaction and effect as evidence of social existence. As a result, the precise relationship between the old body and social identity is obfuscated. Here we show how such bodies both reveal the project which constitutes an individual's past life, as well as providing the material through which that project may be sustained. Whether we are talking of face-lifts, hip replacements or wheelchairs, of elective deafness or selective incontinence, the old body is one which is not only increasingly amenable to 'finishing', but in addition can constitute a powerful social resource.

Chapter 4

Medicalising the body

As accounts of the dead body, each of the descriptions set out below selects and highlights particular aspects of its materiality – its coldness, its discoloration, its disease-ridden nature. Although both *the* body as well as a *particular* body are entirely familiar to the eye of the viewer, death is thought to rob them of that familiarity. These descriptions are therefore implicitly oriented towards a viewer who is not familiar with the appearance and temperature of the dead body. In order to define or describe 'death', its material features have to be spelled out. In this way 'death' can be known:

> Death, signs of: Relaxing of facial muscles, producing rather staring eyes and gaping mouth. Loss of curves of the back, which becomes flat against the bed or table. Slight discoloration of the skin, which becomes a wax-yellow hue, and loses its pink transparency at the finger tips.
>
> > (*Black's Medical Dictionary*, cited in Ball, 1976)

> The cadaver is an object, a repository of disease and infection. It is a container, a shell; at once a solution to a riddle, and an obstacle to knowledge.
>
> > (description of body in mortuary from Prior, 1989)

> Men's bodies 'shattered': the jaws dropped and out poured 'so much blood'. Aeroplane propellers sliced men into pieces. In death, white soldiers turned blackish and black Senegalese soldiers turned whitish.
>
> > (Bourke, 1996)

We sat by her still body in the Intensive Care Unit of the Princess Margaret Hospital in Swindon. She was wired into technology, flawless in her beauty, in spite of the deadly head and chest injuries. The smell of petrol permeated the area around her bed. We held her hand, we prayed...

(Long, 1984)

After she died, I sat with her body, stroking her face, holding her hand. She was cold, and my hand could not warm her hand, But I could not believe that she had stopped breathing: even at the end, she had still been so full of life. Her face looked peaceful; though her eyebrows were raised in a slightly quizzical manner: as if to say, how can this be?

(Picardie, 1997)

These descriptions and definitions have been extracted from a Western social context where the corpse normally lies hidden from the public gaze, visible only under the strictly controlled conditions of the mortuary or Chapel of Rest. As a result, for many viewers, the strangeness of the dead body lies precisely in its materiality, a quality which appears to predominate in the absence of other attributes such as warmth, muscle tone, facial expression and speech. Indeed, it is the body's materiality which must be dealt with as a matter of urgency, lest it smell, produce fluid or infect the bodies of the living (see Chapter 7).

This chapter continues to problematise the ways in which the body is seen to provide crucial evidence as to the nature and status of the self or individual. The materiality of the dead body is, as we show, produced via particular discourses and sets of practices, many of which assume that the corpse stands for, or embodies 'death' (Prior, 1989; Hockey, 1996; Howarth 1996); for example, one of the key texts on bereavement counselling asserts that: '[s]eeing the body of the deceased person helps to bring home the reality and finality of death' (Worden, 1991: 61). Debates as to whether embalming and making-up corpses is, or is not, a 'denial' of death (Huntington and Metcalf, 1979) ride on the assumption that 'death' is a particular set of bodily characteristics which, in being modified, can be made to 'lie'. If those characteristics are transformed or distorted, therefore, 'death' is somehow not quite there – for example, if the colour of the flesh is changed, or if facial features which indicate a fight for breath are massaged into the peaceful indications of a deep sleep (see Chapter 7). This chapter therefore sets out to explore the relationship between perspectives on the dead body, death and the social identities of both the deceased and those who survive them.

First, it is important to recognise the resonance of a view of the dead body which assumes that its material aspects are not only self-evident but also definitive of its status as 'dead'. The idea that 'death' resides in particular material phenomena finds its way, uncritically, into existing social theories of death and the body. As yet there has been little attempt to unpack the culturally specific beliefs and values through which encounters with actual bodies are mediated. For example, in Shilling's comparative account of the work of Berger, Giddens, Bourdieu and Elias, the dead body is taken as a given. Only in its meanings and effects is there any uncertainty or debate. For example, it can be either a threat to meaning, a failed project, lost cultural capital or the limitations of the civilising process (1993: 175–197). Each author has a different take on the significance of the corpse, but none ask how it came to be constituted in the first place, nor wherein the grounds of its materiality might lie. Thus, for Berger, the confrontation with the dead body and therefore one's own mortality is a 'marginal situation' which undermines the apparently objective reality of the human social world and reveals the arbitrariness of culturally-specific meaning systems (cited in Shilling, 1993: 177–189). For Giddens, the dead body is a failed project, a grim reminder that the increasing control which human beings are able to exercise over their bodies is ultimately time-limited (cited in ibid.: 180–185). For Bourdieu, the dead body in high modernity signifies a decline in the individual's symbolic value or capital and therefore a threat to their self identity (cited in ibid.: 185–188). For Elias, the dead body represents problematic evidence of the body's biological, uncontainable and emotive character, despite the civilising processes of socialisation, individualisation and rationalisation (cited in ibid.: 185–188). It is the significance rather than the ontological status of the corpse which concerns these authors, something we also find in connection with the living body. As Armstrong notes, 'sociologists, general and medical, have accepted the body as a given, as the point at which and from which they start their analysis' (1987: 65). Here we suggest that, rather than treating the dead body as a highly unequivocal given, theoretical insight can be enhanced by making the biological 'facts of death' and the dead body a non-self-evident starting point. As Prior says:

> the body is not, and cannot be 'this' or 'that' thing, and it cannot be adequately and fully described by reference to how any one interest group may monopolise and harness its 'properties'. Nor, indeed, is the body something immutable and unchangeable.
>
> (1989: 18)

Professional discourses amplify this point: for example, a text which indicates whether a coroner should investigate a death carries a section entitled: 'What amounts to a body?' (Matthews and Foreman, 1993: 56). It begins by saying that, 'it is necessary to consider first of all what amounts to a body' and signals the problematic hybridity of the following 'corpses': the body of a foetus or stillborn child; old human remains; a partially destroyed body or a part or parts of a body; calcined remains or ashes.

The aim of this chapter is therefore to problematise the event or process we call 'death' and the thing we call a 'dead body'. In this way, our material destabilises any simple, binary opposition between life and death and instead reveals the relationship between body and self and embodied self to be both complex and mutable. The material indicates that the point at which life ends, at which the living individual becomes the dead individual, at which the body becomes the corpse, has never been straightforward. Though it is frequently represented as a self-evident and shocking moment or state – the gasp of horror which confirms that someone is 'dead!' – the ways in which the transition from life to death has been understood vary enormously, both historically and cross-culturally. Arnold and McKee, for example, identify the Western shift from a theological or philosophical discussion as to what and when death might be, to a seventeenth-century scientific debate, one which, in the eighteenth century, became a focus for medical scientists (1997).

Currently, however, there is a common-sense assumption that the dead body has an incontrovertible biological reality which provides us with inescapable, if unpalatable truths about the nature of human life. This notion of the dead body as unmistakably organic is reinforced by the assumption that the individual is no longer present once they have died – they have 'gone' or 'passed away' – and what remains behind is merely flesh and bones, dead meat, a shell or husk, a vile body. That the dead body will deteriorate like other dead matter, such as cut flowers or fresh fish, further bolsters our view of the dead body as a material given. With reference to the living body, Frank highlights the assumption that as a material entity, the body has the capacity to contain truth: 'the enduring belief that the body can provide us with a grounded truth suggests why interest in it should flourish within cultural modernity' (1990: 132). Terry and Urla similarly refer to 'the assumption that bodies, like property, are real material objects whose disposition is of great concern to society as a whole' (1995: 6). They describe the living body as akin to 'all objects that acquire the status of the Real through elaborate processes that present them as material' (ibid.). And it is this materiality, often viewed as the irreducible underpinning of social construction, which, in Butler's view, requires a 'critical genealogy' rather than merely acceptance (1993: 32).

This chapter offers such a genealogy and makes the materiality of the dead body its focus. To this end it highlights the range of technologies through which the apparently irreducible materiality of the corpse is made evident, and problematises the relationship believed to exist between the materialised corpse and death. This is something which may not obtain in other parts of the world. Bloch and Parry (1982), for example, describe the death of the Hindu householder as something which does not take place until the corpse is half-cremated, the point at which the skull is cracked open by the chief mourner and the spirit allowed to escape. Indeed, despite the close association between death and the corpse for Westerners, there remain Western practices which subvert this relationship. Sudnow's (1967) ethnography of the American social organisation of dying in a large, West Coast charity hospital shows how the 'corpse' is made to emerge prior to what is commonly regarded as its 'biological' death. He describes his approach to this study as follows:

> the practices of inspection, examination, disposition, announcing, pronouncing, discharging, wrapping, etc., that I shall explore below, collectively comprise what could be called the 'parent' activity; 'making a dead or dying person'. My emphasis is on the 'production of dying and death'...and on the 'production of a bereaved person'.
>
> (1967: 8)

Sudnow therefore takes the position that if 'death' is the outcome of social practices, then these merit sociological examination and 'death' itself cannot be taken as a given. Thus, on the basis of extensive personal experience, aides in this hospital would predict which patients were about to die. To minimise their contact with death, they would produce a pre-death 'corpse' through practices such as replacing patients' dentures, putting a diaper in place, binding feet and laying a clean sheet underneath them. Once the doctor had officially transformed the 'patient' into a 'corpse' by announcing that death had occurred, all that remained was the wrapping and pinning of the 'dead body'. In this way a pre-death corpse was produced out of the practices of hospital staff (1967). Sudnow's approach to death as something 'produced', via discourses and practices, has proved extremely useful – but it must be recognised that it is not an account of dying as an embodied experience – or an 'unfinished' bodily process (Shilling, 1993). Nonetheless, drawing on Garfinkel's work on procedural definitions (cited in Sudnow, 1967: 9), Sudnow does provide an important and early check on the uncritical use of common-sense categories by sociologists. As he points out, Glaser and Strauss's ground-breaking work on death awareness contexts (1965; 1968) omitted to ask how the category 'dying' was being made to emerge (1967: 62–63).

Here we build upon the view that 'death' cannot be regarded as a straightforward moment or event which coincides with an obvious set of organic changes within the living body. For example, the issue of the body's relationship with, and ultimate separation from the 'soul' has been a long-standing preoccupation of Western philosophers and theologians. Arnold and McKee identify the shift from mechanical identifiers of the presence of life – such as a feather or mirror held to the mouth to trace the presence of breath – to nineteenth century medical instruments which measured the body's functions (1997). Rather than breath alone, respiratory motion, blood flow and the electrical activity of the heart became recordable bodily processes which could be read as evidence of the body's status as either 'dead' or 'living'. As these authors note, the movement of a pen across a rotating drum of graph paper recorded the presence of life; the flat line therefore becoming a representation of death which still survives on monitor screens. More sophisticated technology is often developed in the hope of overcoming these ambiguities, of banishing the hybrid creatures who linger at the boundary between life and death. However, as the issues surrounding stillbirth, persistent vegetative state (PVS) and organ transplantation indicate, this hope has not been realised. In response to the ethical issues which emerge out of transplant surgery, Bartlett (1995) for example, unpacks definitions of death to show that if we think of it as irreversible loss of the organism's integrating function, that is, the loss of function in the cortex, we cannot count events such as cardiac arrest or brainstem death as signifiers of death itself. Though they contribute crucially to the functioning of the cortex, they are causal rather than constitutive of death. Death is therefore identifiable in relation to a particular anatomical region – the cortex. If heart-attack victims are the subjects of Do Not Resuscitate orders, the removal of their organs immediately after cardiac arrest is an act carried out on someone who cannot be categorised as dead. Their condition remains *potentially* reversible.

The associated ethical difficulties bred out of the classification of 'life' and 'death' through quantification or measuring are detailed in Sudnow's ethnography (1967). Here it played a crucial role in allowing interns to assign a status to stillborn infants (ibid.: 109–116). These 'creatures', as Sudnow refers to them, were categorised as either a 'thing', an 'aborted foetus', an 'abortus' or a 'baby' on the basis of their weight, height and length of gestation, a classificatory process which had very specific material outcomes. A few grammes or centimetres determined whether the 'creature' was either flushed down the toilet, bottled or 'admitted to the hospital, wrapped in a morgue sheet, placed in the hospital morgue, and buried in the ground by an authorized burier' (ibid.: 110). Only those who weighed in at above the cut-off point were deemed to have been 'alive' and could, therefore, be said to have 'died'. Contingent upon these few grammes of flesh was also the status of the man and woman responsible for its birth, heavier 'babies' becoming the responsibility of their 'parents' who were then required to arrange and pay for his or her burial.

Specific examples such as these raise more general questions about how the corpse, as an entity, has come into being. Prior argues that Westerners recognise the dead body from marks and signs which are visible on it and in it. Indeed, the Western body becomes a container within which the 'facts, explanations and data on mortality' are believed to reside (1989: 19). He goes on to say that without the corpse, death cannot easily come into being. 'Death', in Prior's terms, is the outcome of a range of social processes – the medical diagnosis of its cause, the registration of a death, grief, preparation for disposal and religious ritual. All these practices, acts and emotional responses are contingent upon the presence of a body which has been categorised as 'dead'. Indeed, as Prior notes, so central is the body to the occurrence of 'death' that body parts such as hands or ashes can sometimes be made to substitute for the whole if matters are pressing. As noted, however, the part-for-whole capacity of the organs is highly dependent upon the social context within which the part is located. For coroners, a body part cannot necessarily stand in for a dead body if it is deemed possible for life to continue without it (Matthews and Foreman, 1993: 56). Simon Armitage (1998) plays on the uncertain part-to-whole nature of the body in a joke about a British prisoner of war who had his successively amputated left arm, right arm and right leg sent back to the United Kingdom for burial. His final request, that his amputated left leg be similarly disposed of, is refused. 'The commandant tells him, "We think you're trying to escape" ' (1998: 81).

Like death itself, grief, as a practice or process which is stimulated by death, is currently seen to be impaired by the absence of the dead body. As a remedy, funerals are sometimes provided in the absence of a body for those individuals and families who have been bereaved through accidents where the body has been either destroyed or lost (Hockey, 1992). This practice reflects the view that grief requires a material focus, and that in the absence of its primary focus – the prepared corpse – ritual time and space can be used to make more tangible that for which there is no material evidence. It is a view which stems from a therapeutic literature on bereavement where, for example, Worden highlights the importance of viewing the body as a way of 'making real the fact of the loss' (1991: 61). It is the body, therefore, which somehow contains the 'truth' about death and much of the bereavement counselling literature concerns itself with the experience of "unreal" death, that is, with death's capacity to somehow "not really happen"' (ibid.: 42). We can argue, therefore, that a set of organic changes such as the cessation of breathing and heart beat do not in themselves add up to 'death', in a Western sense – even though they are integral to its occurrence. For example, 'death' in intensive care is the product of a shift from a mobile to a fixed line on a monitor screen. By contrast, for therapists such as Worden, 'death' is the product of 'work', something which comes into being, in a phenomenological sense, only when the 'tasks' of 'grief work' have been successfully accomplished. First among these tasks is the need 'to come full face with the reality that the person is dead, that the person is gone and will not return' (1991: 10). Without this work, death has no 'reality' – and grief will not ensue. Sudnow's ethnography provides yet another example in that he identifies the work of hospital staff as a set of practices which produce 'death'. And Prior's account of the social organisation of death in Belfast shows 'death' to be the outcome of medical, legal, religious and political activities (1989).

While these Western examples indicate that the materialisation of the dead body is central to the occurrence of 'death', the presence of a corpse may not necessarily be clear, not because its whereabouts are uncertain but rather because its status is ambiguous. Not infrequently, the dead body comes into being only as an outcome of the social relations through which the categorisation of death is negotiated. Thus, the frequent transformation of old bodies into dead bodies which takes place in residential homes is the product of a professional hierarchy which is headed up by a doctor. While matrons and care staff may have extensive experience of the bodies in their care, they cannot 'produce' a corpse independently of a doctor. As Komaromy argues, the category 'dying' is one from which patients are excluded until so categorised by the doctor, a transition which carries the benefits of additional pain relief and other forms of special treatment (Komaromy and Hockey, in press). The position of these care staff is shared by ambulance men. In one case a driver who announced the arrival of a corpse to a waiting casualty doctor was told firmly that the body had no such status or, indeed, reality until so categorised by the doctor. It required the display of the 'patient's' severed head in a bucket by the ambulance driver before his claim to knowledge could be substantiated and the 'patient' could be re-categorised as a 'corpse' – in this case, without the mediating expertise of the doctor (personal communication).

Sudnow's ethnography gives additional evidence of the powerful if problematic role of ambulance men in producing corpses. Here we find ambulance drivers using their sirens to signal that they are carrying a patient/corpse categorised as DOA (Dead On Arrival). Sudnow says that 'the designation "DOA" is somewhat ambiguous insofar as many persons are not physiologically dead upon arrival, but are nonetheless classified as having been such' (1967: 100). As he explains, their subsequent death is often 'back dated' so removing it from the staff's sphere of responsibility. What he goes on to show is that the production of a corpse is intimately linked with the ambulance man's reading of the patient/corpse's social status. Where the patient/corpse is a child or appears wealthy, the signal is louder and more extended, so conveying the message that the body within the ambulance is 'alive' and therefore the medical staff need to be ready for rapid action.

To further discussion of these general points, this chapter provides a more detailed account of two examples which encompass many of the difficulties of defining death and producing the dead body. The first concerns the deaths of individuals who have never engaged in face-to-face social interaction and are not yet seen to have agency, in the more traditional senses of this sociological term. They are babies whose death precedes their birth – or occurs shortly after it. The second example concerns the deaths of individuals who appear able to engage in social interaction, who are not self-evidently without agency and who retain a strong social presence. These are the apparently undamaged people who temporarily 'sleep' on ventilators and other life-support machinery. What we will be examining is the fragile status of the 'lives' and 'deaths' of members of these two social categories. For them, neither the status of their 'life' nor their 'death' has stability, but instead represents the outcome of often competing discursive frameworks and sets of practices. The examples of stillbirth, neonatal death and persistent vegetative state have therefore been chosen because they disrupt the dualistic relationship which currently links both the concepts of 'mind' and 'body', as well as those of 'life' and 'death'.

'Body' and 'death' are currently defined as the negative halves of binary oppositions, their meaning deriving solely from the boundaries or limitations of their positively perceived other halves – 'mind' and 'life'. As Grosz suggests, within dichotomous structures 'one term has a positive status and an existence independent of the other; the other term is purely negatively defined, and has no contours of its own; its limited boundaries are those which define the positive term' (1989: xvi). Within a Western view, therefore, 'mind' is 'correlated with reason, subject, consciousness, interiority, activity and masculinity'. 'Body', by contrast, is 'brute, animalistic, inert, outside of history, culture and socio-political life' (Grosz, 1989: xiv). In the absence of mind, body loses value, its opposite number or defining better half having ceased to be linked with it in any tangible sense. Freed from body, mind, however, continues its existence in the form of its products, reputation and influence. As Grosz says of the positively perceived half of a binary pair: '[it] has an existence independent of the other' (ibid.: xvi) – and indeed we continue to celebrate the 'minds' of Mozart, Shakespeare and Plato long after the demise of their bodies, just as we unknowingly carry forward the beliefs and aphorisms of our long disembodied grandparents.

In a similar fashion, modernity has seen the growing ascendancy of the value of 'life', the positively perceived half of the life/death binary. Its primacy holds sway in the face of an increasingly opaque 'death', often conceived of as void or annihilation. By contrast, sixteenth-century Western religious liturgy reminded believers that 'flesh and blood cannot inherit the kingdom of God'. It gave form to the passage from earthly to heavenly life-after-death through the analogy of sowing seed: 'that which thou sowest is not quickened, except it die'. It is death and not life which causes the seed to 'quicken' into eternal life. That life is the negatively perceived half of this binary is evident:

> [the seed] is sown in corruption; it is raised in incorruption; It is sown in dishonour; it is raised in glory; It is sown in weakness; it is raised in power; It is sown a natural body; it is raised a spiritual body.
>
> (The Book of Common Prayer and Administration of the Sacraments)

Currently, however, 'life' is less a prelude to glory and power and more something to 'live to the full', a 'right' as well as 'the greatest gift'. No longer seen as a 'dress rehearsal', 'life' has now achieved a position of dominance in its own right. Rather than the death of metaphorical seeds, necessary for quickening into eternal life, we are now more concerned with earthly continuities, that is, the sowing of bodily 'seeds' and their long-term survival through the procreative activities of our children. Western grandparenthood is now felt to be under threat from a radically diminished male sperm count and a trend towards childlessness through choice.

Grosz argues that 'dichotomies are inherently non-reversible, non-reciprocal hierarchies, and thus describe systems of domination' (1989: xvi). However, when it comes to the discursive practices associated with stillbirth and persistent vegetative state (PVS), we find that systems of power become destabilised, even though they are elsewhere unchallenged. While it remains the case that we are dealing with difference – what is 'mind' is not 'body'; what is 'life' is not 'death' – the dichotomous and therefore irreversible or non-reciprocal nature of these categories becomes less evident. They are not mutually exhaustive and can admit further terms or categories such as comatose or stillborn. As a result the dominant conceptual differentiation represented by the binary life/death becomes difficult to achieve in practice. Its status is reduced to little more than a hypothesis about the nature of human existence, rather than an incontrovertible reality. In practice, the life/death differentiation may be unsustainable with any ease or clarity. Rather, it constitutes a cultural imperative to differentiate between unstable yet highly valued categories. We find a parallel case in Victorian concepts of sexual difference. Matus challenges the idea that this was an era when sexual differences were clearly understood and experienced as unambiguous (1995). Rather, she argues, medical discourses of the time were much taken up with the problem of sexual ambiguity or slippage. Thus the threat to 'respectable' society posed by 'deviant' categories of women such as prostitutes was framed in terms of hybrid physiological characteristics such as a hoarse masculine voice and morbid ovaries. This may surprise us since sex differences are not ordinarily seen as indeterminate bodily characteristics. Yet when we look in detail at the apparently self-evident differentiation between life and death we find, particularly in examples such as stillbirth and PVS, a similar indeterminacy.

Just as medicine has played a central role in managing nineteenth-century concerns about the unstable boundary between the sexes, so medical categories have been important as a way of establishing life's boundaries, a project which has its roots in the dualistic thinking of eighteenth century scientific world views. This approach has not meant, however, that either the means of measuring, or the nature of that which should be measured, has been obvious or agreed upon. Medical opinions still vary as to which of the body's functions or systems should form the basis of a decision that life has ended, that the living body is now the dead body (Bartlett, 1995). However, this chapter concerns itself not so much with the tensions which are internal to medical science, but rather the way in which, as a framework of ideas and practices, it contributes to the production of death and the dead body in a broader sense. As Illich pointed out: 'The doctor's grasp over life starts with the monthly prenatal check-up when he decides if and how the foetus shall be born; it ends with his decision to abandon further resuscitation' (Illich, cited in Harvey, 1997). It is precisely these two points within the life course, birth and death, which this chapter takes up. Illich's concentration on the doctor's 'grasp over life' reminds us that the body cannot be viewed as a given – but rather as a product. Unlike Illich, however, we here examine the doctor as but one among a number of 'interested parties' who participate in the production of the dead body, though not necessarily in ways which produce a single and agreed upon corpse. Viewed in this way, it becomes evident that a plurality of 'deaths' and 'dead bodies' is often in existence, particularly in the cases of stillbirth and PVS.

Measuring up to life

As discussed, measurement can play a crucial role in the medical categorisation of stillbirth. The issue of abortion, that is the choice to expel the embryo from the uterus and remove any possibility of a future life, raises questions about its status and rights, many of which hinge upon the point at which it can be said to be 'alive'. This lack of clarity makes the unchosen 'death' of the foetus particularly difficult to produce. As Sudnow showed, it is not only difficult to know what has 'died', but also whether it has 'died', since an answer to the paired question – has it lived? – is similarly elusive. Depending upon how it measures up, the 'creature' which is delivered may be assigned the status of a 'thing'. In this case, as Sudnow says, 'it does not move from life to death, as these categories are socially used, but from biological activity to inactivity' (1967: 110). Within the contrasting discursive context of the Catholic Charismatic Church in North America, abortions, miscarriages and stillbirths constitute a single category of *in utero* death, unbaptised infants requiring healing rituals before they can go to heaven (Csordas, 1996: 230–231). An abortion, even more than a stillbirth or miscarriage, is seen as a 'powerful pathogenic agent' which requires the antidote of this ritual. The dead foetus is named, symbolically baptised and so granted the cultural status of a person. The abortion is thus undone. At a subsequent mass the woman is enjoined to let the Eucharist flow through the aborted child and all other dead family members. Csordas contrasts this data with the wealth of ethnographic evidence which shows personhood to be a status often not assumed until well after birth: he says, 'in Charismatic healing a never-to-be-born fetus is still a person' (ibid.: 234). Another indicator of the diversity of discursive contexts within which abortion takes place is legislation. Legally controlled in the United Kingdom only from the nineteenth century, abortion had become totally criminalised by 1861. Only in 1967 were the UK abortion laws relaxed. However, as the medical context changes – making survival possible for babies of only 24 weeks – so the boundary between legal abortion and illegal killing shifts and 24 weeks has become the latest point at which abortion can take place (Pascall, 1997).

Heald with Brown take up these ambiguities in a report on a group called Care for Bereaved Parents, set up in 1990 at South Cleveland Hospitals, Middlesbrough, England (1994). Until the early 1980s, women and men in Middlesbrough who had been bereaved through stillbirth or neonatal death were discouraged from making contact with the body of their baby or indeed dwelling on their loss. Few saw or held the baby's body. In being excluded from social interaction and ritual practices such as a funeral, no 'baby' or indeed 'parent' was actually produced. Waste organic matter had been expelled from a woman's body. If she had no other children, 'parenthood' was merely a future aspiration which she was encouraged to pursue as soon as possible. With the inception of the new service, parents were not only offered counselling but also encouraged to engage in practices which would affirm the human status of their stillborn child, as well as the set of relationships within which it was located. Thus they began to view, dress, cuddle, name, measure and photograph the body of their baby. Rather than organic waste material, to be incinerated or buried in a shared, unmarked grave in hospital grounds, the material body became the locus of identity for the parents' would-be daughter or son.

This personalising of the dead body of the stillborn child stands in marked contrast with the de-personalisation of the living bodies of elderly people. Here the individualising processes of naming and photographing and the interactive practices of cuddling and dressing are less likely to occur. In residential care, for example, the individuality of those who have survived friends and family is not only highly distinctive but can also be problematic. For visiting relatives, the older person who is sick or disabled provides a troubling contrast with their former, remembered self, their changed 'home' and physical and mental circumstances revealing the mutability of human embodiment. For staff, the steady decline and death of the individuals for whom they may have cared across months, if not years, is a challenging confrontation with personal mortality and the transience of all human bonds. As a result, the institutional categories of 'staff' or 'resident' play an important role in submerging the individuality of these particular old people. Encompassed within a social pattern of group living and a rigid temporal structuring of bedtimes, mealtimes and bathtimes, the absence or permanent loss of an individual becomes irrelevant to the daily unfolding of a hierarchical pattern of social categories. Research in a local authority residential home revealed that no visible marker of a resident's presence remained once they had died: their clothing, room and dining room space being rapidly redistributed among other residents (Hockey, 1990: 110). The social identity of older adults living in residential care is therefore increasingly a product of private memories, rather than the outcome of individual embodied performance. Rooted in the past, it exists only to the extent that it can be invoked in residents' oral accounts, their remaining personal possessions, their scars and bodily damage and in the gestures and remarks through which they resist the anonymity of institutional life (ibid.: 127). However, the social identities which are conferred upon the bodies of dead babies through practices such as dressing and naming, derive from an imagined future rather than a remembered past. Retrieved from the projections of parents and others, these externally derived identities are imposed upon the residual flesh of the foetus. This practice contrasts with the more common Western model of the self and its agency having their source and locus within the body (Moore, 1994).

Though these identities stem from the imaginations of parents and are not bounded by specific time frames, the bodies through which these projections are materialised are viable human beings only if they conform to measurable criteria. While the status of Sudnow's 'creatures' was determined by weight and length, time provided the benchmark against which the Cleveland 'babies' were measured, 14 weeks' gestation being the point after which parents would be offered the opportunity to bury or cremate their 'child'. Prior to this, the 'products of conception' would be incinerated within the hospital, though a service was offered as an acknowledgement of the special nature of these fragments.

Temporal frameworks can therefore provide a crucial yardstick which allows life and death to be differentiated in an apparently dualistic manner. However, as noted, stillbirth and neonatal deaths are events which destabilise a simple life/death binary. Lovell, for

example, identifies the role of healthcare professionals in constructing a 'continuum of pregnancy', ranging from miscarriage, through
stillbirth to neonatal death (1997). It is a value-laden continuum
which informs the structuring of a corresponding 'hierarchy of
sadness', supposedly experienced by women who are bereaved in this
way. Placed at the top of the league-table of grief are those parents
bereaved of a child soon after its birth, a loss which attracts far more
professional care and concern than the much commoner experience
of miscarriage. As evidence for this professionally generated
hierarchy, Lovell cites the work of consultant psychiatrist, Emanuel
Lewis, in whose view 'parents of stillborn infants...should be
encouraged to salvage everything they can from the experience...by
contrast...people should not be pushed into magnifying miscarriages (common, one in three or four pregnancies) into tragedies'
(1997: 41). From the findings of Lovell's study, however, there is no
evidence for this gradation of emotion within parents' experience,
whether it is structured by length of gestation or rarity of event.
Instead parents find themselves caught up in a web of medical,
religious, feminist and familial discursive practices which variously
define and redefine the nature of what, or who, has been lost. For
example, while stillbirths require a Document of Stillbirth,
miscarriages do not and indeed can be treated as gynaecological
scrapings (Lovell, 1983). Even among those babies who are stillborn
rather than miscarried, some are disqualified from babyhood on
account of a deformity. As Lovell points out, 'medical professionals
often referred to a stillborn as a "bad baby"... this linguistic
slippage between medical and everyday terms indicated deep-rooted
feelings as to what constituted a baby and what babies "ought" to be
like' (ibid.: 756).

The 'deaths' of babies, whether before or soon after birth, are
therefore the outcome of a range of personal and professional
practices; biological changes within the bodies of infants; the
emotional experiences of the parents; the realignment of kinship
systems; and a range of medical, legal, ritual and bureaucratic
framings of the event. Experienced in combination they may serve
to produce not just one but several 'deaths' and indeed several lives.
Histologists and morticians, for example, pointed out that 'here we
are only interested in the specimen' – as opposed to the baby which
has died or its parents (Heald with Brown, 1994). However, the
introduction of practices which imposed a social identity upon the
'specimen' had impacted upon this category of professionals with

the result that 'now we realise that parents do want to know what is happening' (ibid.: 3, 4). Histologists' role is to determine the medical factors which contributed to the death, using the techniques of post-mortem examination to produce death via a narrative which makes sense of the event.

Morticians also produce a particular kind of death in that their role is to construct the kind of body parents are encouraged to expect. Somehow they must transform the post-mortem remains of the foetus into a 'child' which is sufficiently robust to stay in one piece during parental cuddling and dressing. That parental expectations have produced a demand for some kind of transformation, or production, is evident from the 'magical' metaphors through which they describe their very practical work: 'people come here and they expect us to perform miracles[...]we have no magic solutions in this profession. It is a very difficult area because these babies are so small and so delicate' (Heald with Brown, 1994, 3, 9–10).

In carrying out their work, morticians find both their time and their expertise as professionals jeopardised. The restoration of the foetus after post-mortem examination is a time-consuming task which, as noted, cannot always be accomplished to everyone's satisfaction. Restored through the use of superglue, the body of the foetus may not hold up to parental contact and so call into question the mortician's skills. Further, the work achieved through use of this adhesive can be undone by the embalmer's chemicals, so rendering the work a costly waste of time. Through the agendas and the practices of parents, morticians and embalmers, therefore, different kinds of 'corpse' and different kinds of 'death' are being produced.

There are, however, further divergencies. Alongside the tensions arising out of a clash of professional boundaries can be identified the ambiguities which parents themselves experience in relation to the child. The organisation Care for Bereaved Parents draws on the model of mourning as:

> a dual process of detachment from the loved one that is moderated by identification. The bereaved take into themselves aspects of the deceased, but because a foetus or newborn has not lived long enough as a separate person, the parents have little to take into themselves of their baby.
>
> (Heald with Brown, 1994: 2, 3)

Practitioners seeking to further this 'task' of 'grief work' therefore aim to simultaneously stage a material encounter with 'death' – in its currently accepted form of the dead body; as well as helping to construct a 'son' or 'daughter' which can be identified with or internalised. Parents themselves mirror these ambiguous understandings as to what or who they are encountering when exposed to the dead baby. For example, one woman said:

> In the room I was in [in the hospital], the baby was next door, and they said any time you want to see him, just call us and we'll bring him in for you, and it was lovely the room…it scared me a bit, you know the baby being next door, but then I got used to the idea, I had him in with me all night once.
>
> (Heald with Brown, 1994, 2, 6–7)

The dead body lying in the next room is therefore, at one and the same time, something frightening, especially when in close proximity, and someone to hold close throughout the night. The materiality of this corpse is both decaying matter to be avoided as well as a baby son to be cuddled in the warmth of the bed.

The materialisation of social identity

The cases of miscarriage, stillbirth and neonatal death, when viewed over the last century, provide clear examples of the instability of that which has come to be seen as the irreducible materiality of the dead body. Before 1803, abortion was legal prior to the quickening, the baby's first perceptible movements. Normally felt at about twelve weeks, the quickening was the point that the soul was believed to enter the foetus and the category 'live' was conferred upon it (Lovell, 1983). Its 'death' by abortion could not therefore take place before it had become 'alive'. Currently medical rather than religious definitions shape the responses of survivors, both professional and lay, to the dead infant. In both cases, however, it the measurement of time which allows the living foetus to be differentiated from the 'products of conception'. Time therefore provides a framework or filter through which the contents of the womb are read. Alongside discursive classificatory systems, whether of a medical or religious nature, we consider the 'productive' role of social practices. Thus, religious and social ritual practices may determine whether or not dead babies are thrown away or burned.

Van Gennep ([1909] 1960) notes that it is the failure to baptise infants who subsequently die which denies them the status of being fully 'alive', rather than their measurement against medical criteria which distinguish 'live' from 'still' births. Without an appropriate ritual practice, there is in principle no transition into the category 'alive'. Through ritual, therefore, 'life' is imposed upon the womb's products, rather than discursively read out of them. While the meaning of such practices may have changed, among contemporary medics, dead infants still have only a fragile toe-hold as social beings. Those born with deformities are 'the monsters...they're disgusting. They should be destroyed...wiped off the face of the earth (Doctor J.)'. And even those born without deformities may still be seen as more fitted to heavenly realms than human society: 'he's beautiful...too beautiful for this world (midwife)' (Lovell, 1983: 756–757).

In the example of pre- or neonatal death a circularity becomes apparent in that medical science, as a framework of ideas and practices, not only draws on, but also constitutes and contributes to the social production of death and the dead body. And indeed, in practice, as Lovell's material indicates, there is a marked slippage between the lay and specialised language through which the death of the infant comes into being (1983). In many cases the stillborn or neonatal body may not resemble anything that has ever lived, either because it is 'monstrously' deformed or because it has become macerated – partly decomposed – while in the womb.

Touch was the sense which initially allowed the 'quickening' to be identified as the point at which the foetus became alive. Currently, sight has gained precedence as a more precise means of identifying the presence of 'life', in that technology now allows a medical 'gaze' to be introduced into the womb via the ultra-sound scanner. Instead of needles swung over the swollen abdomen, grainy photographic images are the means by which the baby's sex, for example, may be detected. The production of the 'live' foetus, whether through touch or sight, is therefore a complex social process, the result being that its 'death' can remain elusive and variously understood.

The relationship between body and self

We now move on to the example of the body which is 'alive' only by virtue of technological support. The body of the dead infant stands in stark contrast with the brain dead or comatose body which has entered a persistent vegetative state (PVS). While the parents of dead babies may strive to impose an externally generated social 'life' and identity upon the remnants of their child, the contrastingly 'lifelike' appearance of the comatose individual serves to sustain 'life', along with the pre-existing set of social relations within which it has unfolded. For relatives, therefore, the brain dead individual's previous social status as 'alive' persists into the present, with the result that the switching-off of a ventilator and the surgical removal of an organ represent the killing and subsequent violation of a 'son', 'daughter' or 'spouse'. Despite high profile campaigns to promote organ donation and the construction of the dead donor as hero, Robbins reports that the rates of refusal to donate 'stubbornly persist at around the 30 per cent level' (1996: 183). In some cases, however, the transplantation of organs from the brain dead but ostensibly living body, into the sick body of another, can provide a sense of continuity. This apparently contrasting response in fact reflects a similar underlying sense of the 'life' of the relative persisting into the present and indeed into the future. For example, the sister of a donor said: 'Oh. it's great because part of Kevin is still going on' (Robbins, 1996: 184). Should the recipient's body fail to accept the organ, a subsequent bereavement may be experienced (Komaromy and Hockey, in press). We can make a contrast between this symbolic identification of the person with particular organs and the coroner's more functional dismissal of 'inessential' body parts such as limbs. They do not of themselves constitute a 'body' which merits an inquest (Matthews and Foreman, 1993). Among the donor families, certain body parts are also seen as less 'essential' to the integrity of the deceased – though here their 'essence' is more to do with person or personality than body function. Eyes, for example – the windows to the soul – may be considered a more 'costly' donation than kidneys or hearts.

Robbins' argument reveals that the medical practice of organ transplant and the responses of donor's relatives expose the production of more than one body and indeed more than one death in the case of the coma victim. Thus medics encounter the PVS patient via the metaphor of the body as machine. This is evidenced in the language of 'extracting', 'salvaging' and 'replacing' organs, a core medical framing of the body which is supported and reinforced by subsidiary notions of the body as an ecological resource which can be recycled as part of a larger biomass – with the result that organs are 'harvested' or 'retrieved'. Medics also construct the PVS body as a gift which is owned by the individual and subsequently their family; its organs can therefore be 'donated', 'gifted' and 'received'. Congruent with this model is also the notion of the body as a commodity from which organs can be 'procured' and, in some countries, exchanged for financial reward (Robbins, 1996).

Each of these models reveals the centrality of the Cartesian mind/body split within the medical management of PVS and organ transplantation. The body itself is ultimately an object which the individual, as a separate entity, can choose to give away after death, in part or in its entirety. Whether the individual is seen to be annihilated at death or whether they are believed to survive in another form or another realm, the centrality of the mind/body split means that the body itself is neither necessary to, nor constitutive of, the individual. The medical body is therefore one which the individual has, rather than is (Csordas, 1994: 53). This view informs the practices of doctors but it is not necessarily shared by relatives or individuals contemplating carrying a donor card. Robbins describes families' 'multi-layered concoction of religious, quasi-religious, and superstitious beliefs that contradict the mind/body dichotomy and assert that the body is more than simply the sum of its physical parts' (1996: 191). It is therefore, as she argues, an embodiment of the dead individual and all that they stood for – rather than a separate object possessed by that individual.

Unstable binaries

The examples of the stillborn baby and the PVS patient highlight a more widespread lack of consensus at to what constitutes the dead body. The material discussed above reveals the production of multiple 'dead bodies', each one having a different temporal, spatial and social location. Flesh is variously read; variously attributed with the status 'alive' or 'dead'; variously understood in terms of its relationship with the individual. Once the apparently irreducible materiality of the dead body has been destabilised, other 'truths' become similarly questionable; for example, the notion that the 'reality of death' resides within the dead body. In therapeutic theory it is the encounter with the corpse which provides relatives with overwhelming evidence that their father's or husband's or daughter's life is over. Yet, as discussion of pre-natal or neonatal 'death' indicates, that 'dead body' may provide the substance through which a daughter or son's social life can be made to begin; and conversely, the 'living' bodies of very elderly people may not constitute sufficient of a resource for resisting the 'social death' which younger adults impose upon older adults in response to the extreme physical and mental frailty of the old body. One further paradox, however, lies in the area of touch, something seen as a way of conferring social identity upon frail babies, yet confined to those infants whose condition hospital staff have already diagnosed as terminal. The handling of such babies may therefore bring them alive in a social sense; but it simultaneously affirms their status as 'dying' (Symon and Cunningham, 1995; Young, 1997; Crombie, 1997). In later chapters we go on to examine 'lives' lived entirely in the absence of a body. Not only does it become difficult therefore to identify 'death' and link it straightforwardly to a 'dead' body, but the differentiating boundary between 'life' and 'death' itself becomes highly problematic.

The dead body is therefore a signifier which, variously and temporarily, has meant 'the end of life'; 'death'; 'an embodiment of the individual'; 'the absence of the individual'. However, depending upon the discursive context within which that dead body is located, different meanings will be attributed to it. We can therefore challenge 'the enduring belief that the body can provide us with a grounded truth' (Frank, 1990: 132), and instead recognise that the truth 'intrinsic' to these bodies is highly precarious. That 'alive' and 'dead' may each be a status which is constructed rather than grounded in any kind of ineluctable material reality is a position which we have to consider. Sausurrean linguistics highlights the meaning-giving capacity of binary oppositions (see Weedon, 1997). Like the mutually defining relationship between 'man' and 'woman', the definitions of 'life' and 'death' emerge out of their opposition to one another. As noted earlier, however, it is an opposition which no longer carries the same powerful meanings with which it was imbued during an age of religious faith. In the discursive context of Christian liturgy, 'death' signifies the glorious, waiting world of spiritual life, the dominant half of the life/death binary. In more secular contexts, however, where medical science enjoys a position of privilege, 'death' has shifted to a position from which it signifies all that life is not, its shadow side of vulnerability, pain and the ultimate loss of individuality.

What the material presented in this chapter demonstrates is how frequently the binary nature of dominant, often medicalised conceptions of 'life' and 'death', is disrupted. As Matus argues with reference to the male/female binary during the Victorian period, a strongly consensual view conceals a pervasive concern with the possibility of sexual ambiguity or slippage, the merger of that which should be different (1995). In the case of Victorian sexuality, that concern, she stresses, represents a form of control, a representation or indeed re-affirmation of sexuality as it ought to be. While life and death, like male and female, might seem to be all too natural distinctions, we would argue here that it is an over-determined binary which reflects an underlying concern with slippage between the two categories. The fear of being buried alive inspired the early use of feathers and mirrors to detect the presence of breath. That life should be clearly distinguishable from its negative, shadow half – death – is also an imperative which stalks the corridors of residential homes (Hockey, 1990). Within the biological continuum of human physical and mental deterioration, boundaries and distances are introduced, such that the 'fit' are required to conform to a rigid structuring of mealtimes, bathtimes and bedtimes while the 'frail' are confined to sick bays, the 'frail' corridor and easy-access seating alcoves well within sight of staff. Those who are believed to have made an irreversible transition to the category 'frail' may, like neonatally deceased children, yield up their personhood and take on the status of 'vegetable', 'little doll' or 'puppet'. On a social level, at least, they have already died.

Conversely, as later chapters detail, the return and particularly the ambulant return of the dead, similarly haunt the imagination across time and culture, whether in the form of zombie, vampire or ghost. Du Boulay (1982) provided an account of the patterning of death ritual in rural Greece which pervades both dance and the organisation of marriage. Failure to adhere to this pattern can provoke the return of the dead in the form of a vampire, a belief which, she reports, was no mere folk tale but one which older members of the community recollected as an actual event. In the residential home, the presence and potential presence of the dead also preoccupy staff. Throughout each night they monitor sleeping residents, reaffirming their status as 'alive' on an hourly basis. Even during the day, the very shallow breathing of a resident who napped on her bed raised concern among staff on more than one occasion. Had she made an unscheduled transition to the category 'dead'? In break-time chat, staff rehearse their concern about slippage between the social and institutional categories: 'alive' and 'dead'. For example, referring to a recently deceased resident, a care assistant asked Deputy Matron: 'Has Mrs Atkinson been coffined?'. Only later was the Deputy Matron able to laugh about her own horror, inspired by her misinterpretation of the word 'coffined': 'Has Mrs Atkinson been coughing?'. The return to 'life' of residents laid out in the home's mortuary was therefore a not infrequent source of anxious joking. A domestic claimed that the body of a particular resident was not in the mortuary when she cleaned it and staff teased her that the resident had popped out to the toilet. When staff found the morgue doors flapping open one morning they told one another shock horror fantasies of corpse and trolley rolling out into the courtyard and away down the drive (Hockey, 1990).

Grosz (1989) describes binaries as mutually exhaustive categories, the subordinate half representing everything that the dominant is not. Yet in the material presented here, the limits of one category cannot be so easily differentiated from the limits of the other. Death can be partial, for example, as evidenced in the case of social death, so providing the substance of a hybrid, third category. In November 1996, 53-year-old Ramon Sempedro, paralysed from the neck down for 28 years, described himself to a Spanish court as 'a living head on a dead body'. In a strongly Roman Catholic society, only 60 per cent of the population would support euthanasia in cases such as this. Indeed, Luis de Moya, priest, academic and quadriplegic, re-ascribed valuable human agency to living-head-on-a-dead-body Ramon Sempedro: 'Given his talents, there is a great deal he could do, especially helping other people in similar circumstances' (*The Guardian*, 14 November 1996). In a bodily sense, therefore Mr Sempedro is both – and neither – 'alive' and/nor 'dead'. Having become a *cause célèbre*, his 3-year-long unresolved legal battle for assisted suicide positioned him within an autonomous category and set him apart from the binary, 'life'/'death'. In 1995, Jean-Dominique Bauby, editor-in-chief of French *Elle*, suffered a similar experience when he was totally paralysed by a massive stroke. Only the fluttering of one eyelid remained to him as a means of communication. Mentally intact, the changed state of Bauby's body leads him to describe the 'snuffing out' of the life he once knew (1997: 11). Known as 'locked-in syndrome', his condition is poorly understood since, as he says, 'most victims are abandoned to a vegetable existence' (ibid.: 19). Alongside those who might be categorised as either the 'living' but socially dead or the physically deceased but undead, there are other human embodiments which disrupt binary classificatory systems. Limbs, long incinerated, continue to haunt the bodies and selves of those who they, in part, once constituted. Residual hair, ashes, clothes, bones, eyelashes, handwriting, even traces of perspiration and perfume can take on and sustain a 'life' to which they might seem to bear only an iconic relationship. Pilgrims throughout the ages have laboured the routes to the remaining fragments of the bodies of saints (Geary, 1986).

Not only can the categories 'life' and 'death' be difficult to differentiate from one another in practice, for example, in the case of very elderly people living in residential care, they can also be made to transgress their mutual boundary with the result that additional categories may be constituted. Vialles (1994) provides an example of a similar transgressive move. Her ethnography of an abattoir describes the additional category which emerges within the life/death transition which produces the edible from out of the animal. Abattoirs are the site, or as Vialles says, the 'no-place' within which animals are killed prior to being eaten by human beings. However, she argues that this transformation must occur not just at a material but also, crucially, at a cultural level. Examining both the spatialising as well linguistic processes which make up the killing of an animal, she notes that the term abattoir derives from the word *abattre*, meaning 'to bring down that which is standing'. *Tuer*, meaning 'to kill', is not used in the slaughterhouse. There is a legal requirement to stun animals before slaughter. Once unconscious, they are suspended. Then they are bled. In this way, she argues, a dissociation is introduced between the shedding of blood and the administering of death: 'Who kills the animal? The person who stuns it, or the person who bleeds it?' (Vialles, 1994: 45). After stunning, the animal ceases to be. De-animalisation occurs with suspension. As Vialles says:

> Between the moment of death and the final presentation of the carcass there is a nameless void: the object is neither an animal, nor even (especially not even) a dead animal (a corpse, unfit for consumption), nor is it yet meat.
>
> (1994: 44)

Conclusion

This chapter began with a summary of theoretical orientations towards the concept of 'death', each of which took the dead body as its primary analytic focus (Shilling, 1993). Whether as failed project or lost cultural capital, that body took on a universal and non-problematised relationship with death. This chapter has argued that a more nuanced understanding of the dead body can be derived from an approach which takes as its focus the diversity of dead bodies. Furthermore, in the examples selected, the chapter revealed the often ambiguous status of particular bodies – the stillborn, very elderly, comatose, paralysed and animal body. From this starting point, it becomes possible to ask a series of questions not only about the relationship between 'life' and 'death', but also about the signifying role of bodies, 'alive', 'dead', 'present', 'absent', in relation to the concepts of 'life' and 'death'. As we have shown, bodies can survive the individual, whether as unwanted remains in a sick bay and morgue, or sought-after relic in shrine and altar. Bodies which, in material terms, are thought to be 'still', or stillborn, have emerged as highly mobile in a semiotic sense. Further, to categorise the dead body as 'still' is a discursive practice which is at odds with the phenomenology of the body itself. A physiological examination reveals that the dead body is anything but still. Changes in its temperature, the build-up of gases and the gradual discoloration of particular regions provide crucial components within coroners' narratives about the events leading up to death. The dead body and social identity therefore emerge as entities which, while at times intimately entwined, the latter potentially embodied within the former, are also highly separable, the focus of multiple, often competing discourses and practices.

Chapter 5

Narratives of the body I

The coroner's court

In previous chapters we have argued that the body stands in a more complex relationship with the production and experience of social identity than many theorists have acknowledged. In this and the following chapter we present two case studies, one contemporary and one from the early modern period, both of which provide detailed accounts of social negotiations taking place at the site of the dead body. Via readings of the body in life, each of these cases demonstrates how retrospective interpretations are made as to the cause, circumstances and nature of the death which has taken place. They provide clear insight into the ways in which changes in the body, which might seem unequivocal – the living body is now dead – are, in reality, open to processes of intense negotiation and indeed contestation. In both cases, we see social hierarchies based on gendered and professional sources of power in operation. Beginning with this chapter, we provide a detailed case study of the workings of the coroner's court, based on a study begun in 1993 of the coroner system in three distinct geographical regions of England. Data were collected through in-depth interviews with coroners, their officers, police officers, bereaved families, and other expert and lay witnesses. Lengthy courtroom observations were also undertaken (Howarth, 1997: 145). This is then set alongside the following chapter's historical material which provides an analysis of witnesses' accounts from the Church courts in Canterbury between 1580 and 1640 (Hallam, 1994). These accounts were recorded in court during the proceedings of legal action, taken when wills were disputed, and, as we go on to show, contained detailed descriptions of the deathbed since it was regarded as the most important site for confirming the last wishes of the person.

Throughout England and Wales, and indeed in many other Western societies, sudden death requires investigation by the coroner or a similar officer. Here the corpse is central to the (re)construction of the self. Unlike the medical body (see Chapter 4) which is ambiguous in that the question of whether it is alive or dead is open to dispute, the body which falls within the coroner's jurisdiction is irrefutably dead. Yet, while it holds the key to a variety of meanings and narrative constructions of the lost self, this does not mean that the dead body is an unambiguous entity; rather, it remains a focus for discourse and practice.

Bodies are sites of struggle over definitions over what is deemed normal and what deviant. Moreover, as Terry and Urla note, 'the notion that individuals identified as socially deviant are somatically different from "normal" people is a peculiarly recurring idea that is deeply rooted in Western scientific and popular thought' (1995: 1). In the context of the coroners' system, the corpse is the material object over which individuals and groups contest a biography for the deceased, defining natural and non-natural death, deviant and non-deviant life-styles, order and disorder in society. Whilst knowledge produced about a particular death situates the body within a professional or personal chronology, it may also point to a broader social disorder. The knowledge ceded by the dead body may not only explain the death and the final stages of the deceased person's life, it may also contain signs of, and clues to another act, as in the case of homicide, where the marks of traumatic death that are found on, around and within the body represent a wider disorder.

As with medicine, and other dominant discourses, the investigation into sudden death begins with the body; it is from the corpse that it derives its knowledge of life. The uncertainty in relation to the suddenly dead body is the unknown story which preceded the death. Because the corpse is silent, inert and therefore open to the production of meaning, that story is discursively constituted by others rather than self-constructed by the individual. This narrative is produced at the inquest from a medley of knowledge bases or discourses – ranging from family, friends and colleagues' immediate experience of the individual to the objective testimony of the expert. The body itself provides the material evidence of the life that was lived, but has a multi-dimensional quality, interpretations of which fall into two broad frameworks and act to produce two bodies: the medico-legal body and the social body. Each of these frameworks defines the corpse as a source of knowledge. In the hands of experts employing scientific methods, the body is made to yield medical and legal truths about death. For the families, although the body continues to be a subject, a person, it is, nevertheless, surveyed and interrogated to assist survivors in the reconstruction of an ongoing biography and identity for the deceased and in turn to adjust their own self-perception. Changes in the self-identity of the deceased, produced at the time of the inquest, can have powerful implications for the identities of close survivors. As noted in Chapter 1, the Western notion of the self as unitary or bounded is a specific and limited formulation of social identity. In the wider repercussions of a coroner's verdict upon the 'selves' of survivors, we see that a particular self cannot be conceived of as 'closed, autonomous or impermeable' (Battersby, 1993: 38).

In the process of interrogating the body, therefore, multiple identities or selves appear, each produced because different readers have different purposes and agendas; family, friends, pathologists, the police, health and safety officials, insurance inspectors, and so on. Biographies are contested and tensions arise between differing accounts. The conflict of perceptions is not solely between scientific and popular accounts of the death. Sudden death, especially when it occurs in early or mid-life, may result in disputes between relatives and friends as to its nature and cause. Among the bereaved, there may be different interpretations of the death as each stands in a distinct relation to the deceased. Diverse knowledge claims carry different weight: expert knowledge asserts dominance over lay accounts. Intimate or lay knowledge also reflects hierarchies as a mother or lover may believe themselves to hold greater insight into the death than, for example, a sibling or friend. Harmonious accounts of the death can only be achieved if the expectations of all interested parties are analogous. In a discussion of bereavement, Walter (1996) describes the manner in which the friends of a deceased woman together produced a biography of her life with which they were all content. In that situation it must be assumed that in the production of her story they shared a common purpose and broadly similar bases for knowledge – creating or recreating a character that fitted their social needs. In other words the individual's relationship to the body – whether object or subject – and their relationship to the deceased person, will influence the meaning and life-commentaries which each derive from it. In the particular crisis of sudden death, the scope for retrospective biographies which are in tension with one another is, however, enormously increased. Much may hinge upon a particular account; for example, the status of professional and parental reputations, the risk of claims for damages, the value attached to marital fidelity. It is a situation in which families and friends often reassess or reconstruct their own identities in response to the body of the deceased. Damage limitation may be high on a number of agendas. By contrast, experts are projecting their professional authority in relation to the object body, clearly distinguishing and marking out the boundaries between themselves and the corpse. As experts they have no living knowledge of the body that confronts them; it has only been known in death. Yet while this process may succeed in distancing the expert from the deceased, it can simultaneously intensify the emotional involvement of the family, for example, as their reaction to hearing the content of the pathologist's report, often for the first time, creates anew the horror of the death.

It is the role of the coroner to translate the diverse accounts in such a way as to piece together the jigsaw of the end of life. The coroner has the ultimate power to interpret the various readings and to translate the social discourse of lay witnesses, replete with subjective observations and common-sense knowledge, into a knowledge about death which fits an objective legal verdict. Coroners must define the nature of death, and give form to the once lost, and now reconstructed self. In so doing, they create the distinction between the dead and the disposable body – the former only becoming the latter once it has given up its knowledge.

This chapter focuses on the coroners' system as one vehicle for exploring the cultural and social processes through which meanings and interpretations are constructed at the site of the dead body. It begins with a discussion of what constitutes a dead body and then provides a brief explanation of the work of the coroners in investigating sudden, unexpected death. It then continues with a discussion of the different readings taken from the body and shows how these are constituted from either scientific or popular discourse. As we will show, tensions between different readings are brought to the fore during the inquest where coroners struggle to recreate a social being recognizable to all. Just as medical knowledge and expertise are based on the dead body, laid out in the dissecting room, so too the coroner's investigation takes the body itself as its starting point. Coroners then employ knowledge from internal and external examinations to look back and make sense of the life that preceded the death.

What is a dead body?

Coroners cannot conduct an inquiry into death unless a dead body is found within their district. What is sometimes unclear, however, is what constitutes a 'dead body'. In the majority of cases, inquests are held on complete human bodies, whether fully grown adults or newly born babies. There are certain categories of body, though, which impel the coroner to pose the question, 'what amounts to a body'? (Matthews and Foreman, 1993) This is usually asked of body fragments where, in considering the wholeness of the body, there is a need to establish whether missing parts could mean that the person is still alive. For example, in case where limbs have been found but no torso. Similarly, a problem arises in the case of calcined remains or ashes where the coroner must verify that these are human remains and, furthermore, that there is a sufficient quantity to constitute a body.

A further category of dead matter that needs to be clarified is the body of a foetus or stillborn baby. We have already considered the ambiguities of the foetus or stillborn body in the preceding chapter. For the coroner, however, distinguishing it as a dead body hinges on its viability outside the mother's womb. Relying on the binary division between life and death, if the body can be shown never to have lived outside its host body, then it cannot claim the status of living and so cannot be classified as dead.

There is a further category of ambiguous body. Consider the following case.

> On the evening of the 8th of May 1950 a man's naked body was unearthed in Tollund Fen, Bjaeldskov Dal, Denmark. The farm workers who found him immediately alerted the local police. The man had suffered a violent death. A rope was clearly visible encircling his neck with the noose drawn tight around his throat. Although slightly decomposed, the body was substantially whole. His hair, worn under a cap, was short and he had short stubble on his upper lip, chin and cheeks. His eyes were closed and his lips partly so. Most of his upper body was still covered with skin. His sexual organs were intact. Internal examinations revealed that his head and brain were undamaged and the fact that his wisdom teeth were largely developed suggested that he was well over 20 years of age. The post-mortem found that his internal organs were sound. The contents of his

stomach revealed that his last meal had comprised of some form of gruel consisting of vegetables and pulses and had been eaten between 12 and 24 hours prior to his death.

(Glob, 1977)

In this case the man was found to be over 2000 years old, his body well preserved by the peat bog in which he had lain for that period. In these circumstances, despite the violent nature of the death, there was no requirement for an inquest. 'In practice the coroner is unlikely to consider an inquest necessary in the case of a discovery of anatomical specimen or in a case where the death must have taken place a long time ago' (Matthews and Foreman, 1993: 57). Within the framework of the coroner's discursive practices, the relics of the dead can therefore be shifted from the category 'dead bodies' and be transformed into anatomical curiosities or objects of fascination. Although the material features of this man's body provided ample evidence of the social life he had led – for example, what he had eaten for his last meal – and medico-legal experts were able to shed light on the nature and cause of his death, for the purposes of the coroner his body did not constitute a 'dead body'. Rather, with the passage of time it had become an archaeological object. There were no relatives, friends or associates remaining to recognise him, but, moreover, outside a museum there was no social context in which to place him within contemporary Western society. Falling outside the discourses through which the social body is produced, he became a clinical object, a focus for scientific interrogation, an objectified ornament of antiquity. The Tollund Man, as he is now known, lies in a glass case in the Museum of Silkeborg.

The coroner

The social significance of sudden death is that is threatens chaos: the notion that death may be random suggests lack of control. The ordered public ritual of the inquest, with its aim of classifying and explaining mortality, lends death a structured and more predictable veneer. The role of the coroner is to determine who the deceased was, how, when and where s/he met their death. Investigating these factors the coroner is required to take 'public interest' into account. This is defined as having five fundamental features. First, the medical cause of death must be determined, and second, any rumours or suspicion surrounding the death are to be allayed.

Third, the inquiry is to draw attention to the existence of circumstances or conditions, which might give rise to further deaths. Fourth, is the advancement of medical knowledge. Finally, the inquest should seek to preserve the legal interests of the deceased person's family, heirs and other interested parties (Brodrick Committee Report, 1971). If there is suspicion that the death may be unlawful and subject to criminal proceedings, the coroner will open the inquest and, after identifying the deceased and stating his intention to pass the case on to the Criminal Prosecution Service (CPS), close it immediately to await the outcome of the criminal case. What we are describing is therefore a hierarchy of resort, more predictable deaths being made sense of via the informal discussions of friends and family and the 'formality' of the GP's death certificate. Sudden deaths can be 'explained' by coroners, but the complexities of deaths at the hands of others must be unravelled by the CPS.

To achieve the aims of the coroner's court, and to properly identify the deceased and the circumstances of death, it is the dead body which becomes the focus of attention; the starting point for the narrative reconstruction of life. Without a dead body there can be no inquest. As noted in the preceding chapter, the body, whether alive or dead, is seen to provide us with 'grounded truth' (Frank, 1990: 132). The corpse is therefore central to this narrative and it is from the readings of the body of the deceased that the reconstruction begins. Locating the body in time and space, it thus becomes the *fons et origo* of knowledge, the coroner relying on experts to use their medical and legal tools to map the causes of death onto the body. As a source of knowledge the corpse is surveyed for signs and causes of death, examined both internally and externally to yield information about the nature of death, and to set this in the context of the habits and features of life.

During the inquest the coroner calls two distinct types of witness; the expert providing medical and legal evidence, and the lay witness who contributes to the social discourse on death. It is intended that these two forms of testimony will combine to impart a clear sense that the circumstances surrounding the death came together in such a way as to point, unequivocally, to the occurrence of death. On the basis of this understanding, an agreement is produced that it could have been no other way, the death could not have been avoided. Each movement, each action, all behaviour led up to the fatality. Yet, in another sense, it is one of the purposes of the coroner's office to look for factors that may have made it otherwise. In the 'public interest' coroners are tasked with investigating how a death might have been avoided, for example, by a change in the speed limit on a road. At this level, death is an event that need not have occurred.

The medico-legal body

During the inquest, once a lay witness – normally a family member – has fulfilled the legal requirement of identification, the pathologist's report will provide a medical explanation of death. The post-mortem on which this is based begins with an external inspection of the body, searching particularly for signs of natural diseases, demonstrated, for example by skin rashes or swellings; signs of assault; and for traces of poison or other foreign materials. The internal examination which ensues comprises the opening of all cavities and the weighing and dissection of the organs found therein. Blood or tissue samples may be taken for further examination.

It was in the eighteenth century that the body came to be treated 'as something docile that could be subject, used, transformed and improved' (Foucault, 1973: p93). This new approach, which viewed the body as a machine, was central to the development of biomedicine. It was the spread of anatomy and the science of pathology that confirmed the opinion that disease was grounded in the body, its discovery facilitated via internal examination. From this perspective, life is encoded in death. Just as biomedicine begins its search for health via the dissection of the corpse, so the medical pathologist searches the dead body in order to discover the disease or injury which resulted in death. The dead body is a site of knowledge, readings of which lead back to life. The pathologist assumes that the corpse is a site of truths, self-evident truths of death and disease; employing scientific methods, these can be read from the body surfaces and, more significantly, its internal sites. The body thus becomes a container of knowledge for explaining death.

The testimonies of these professionals are based on the narrative of their expert reports – documents which adopt the scientific language of medicine and are perceived by the court as inherently objective, learned and scientific. Yet the information gathered by these examinations of the cadaver does not produce self-evident truths as it requires interpretation by experts well versed in translating bodily signs into values and meaning. Deciphering the significance of weights, measurements, fractures of the bone, changes in organic material, and so on, the scientist 'inscribes and projects powerful cultural meanings' onto the body (Terry and Urla, 1995: 6). The medico-legal body, the site of scientific discourse of the causes and nature of death, is a cultural object, itself the product of classificatory systems (Armstrong, 1983). The language of disease exists within specific cultural contexts and each culture prescribes what is normal and what is deviant (Agich, 1983). As Turner contends, disease is 'a system of signs which can be read and translated in a variety of ways' (1996: 200). In the courtroom the expert discourse carries greater weight than lay interpretations. It is only by virtue of the ideological dominance of scientific discourse in modernist societies, however, that the pathologist's report acquires a centrifugal status around which all other narratives revolve.

The inquest will progress in the light of the pathologist's report, paying particular attention to how the deceased may have come by the injuries evident on the body. Further expert and lay witnesses will be called to set this report into context and to reconstruct the end stages of the life of the deceased. These testimonies retain significance because death is not simply a physiological phenomenon located in the body – it is also read and interpreted by a whole range of other mechanisms, for example, signs such as lack of speech, a line on a monitor, the turning off of a machine, or a lack of news.

The social body

In the inquest into the death there are two agendas or tasks running in parallel. The families seek answers to their questions as to how the death could have occurred. They also require details of the lost time before death in order to compose the last stage of the deceased's biography and to map that narrative onto their own continuing biographies. In contrast, the coroner seeks closure. With an eye to a future existence without the deceased, bereaved people look for explanation, understanding and even compassion, but not necessarily closure.

The family and friends of the deceased need to explain the death – not only to define it as natural or non-natural – but to explain or make sense of separation; to be able, in some way, to put the dead away or to locate them in an appropriate place within their own biographies. This is sometimes interpreted as a need to know that they are dead. In cases of sudden or unexpected death, it is common for there to be a time lapse between last communication with the person and the current knowledge that the person is now dead. In cases of sudden death, bereaved people frequently ask themselves when they last saw the person. What were the key elements of the interaction? What could have happened to explain the death? How should they now locate the dead person in their lives, or, how can they mentally transform the living person into the dead person?

The family have a distinct knowledge of the body of the deceased, often an intimate knowledge, having known the person in life. Accordingly, in their readings of the body and their interpretations of the expert readings, they have an agenda which diverges from that of the professional. The families, however, are severely hampered in their attempts to use the body of the deceased as a source of information and meaning. Following unexpected death, the coroner has a right to possession of the body for the purposes of the inquiry. The coroner also determines when the body may be disposed of. In order to fulfil the duties of the post, the coroner may need to retain the body until a post-mortem has been conducted. In cases of homicide or other unlawful deaths, the body may remain in their custody until the person accused of the killing has obtained a further post-mortem examination.

To all intents and purposes the bereaved have been divested of the body of someone who, to varying degrees, they once 'possessed'. The loss of the body is therefore highly problematic as it is the material remains of the person they knew and as such it holds important memories, connotations and meanings for them. It is also especially significant in trying to understand and come to terms with the death. Survivors, particularly close kin, may need to explore the body's surfaces for signs of damage, to become familiar with the changes to the body in death, and also in viewing, or perhaps holding or cradling the body, to re-establish a previous intimate connection between bodies. Although the physical presence of the dead body may in itself be disturbing, it is nevertheless familiar and, more significantly, sacred to the bereaved. For family and friends, the corpse is not an object, nor is it profane. Distressing as it may be – and it may have become damaged and deformed in death – for them it is not the material remains of the person, but the person themself. The identification process, however, may be the only opportunity for the bereaved to get close to the cadaver. Under these circumstances, however, they are normally instructed not to touch or interfere with the body in any way.

If the family were absent when death occurred, then their first encounter with the body of the deceased may take place in the public mortuary – located in the hospital or attached to the coroner's premises. Legislation requires that the deceased must be identified and this is usually carried out by the next-of-kin or other close family member capable of recognising the body. 'Jervis', the coroner's handbook (Matthews and Foreman, 1993), refers to some of the problems and difficulties in identifying certain bodies. For example, the body may have been disfigured by the nature of death; it may have lain for some considerable time and be in a state of decomposition. Wherever possible, however, relatives will be relied upon to make the initial identification.

There is tension in this process. For the professionals who have taken custody of the body it is a corpse, an object, which, for identification purposes can be described according to its facial features, height, weight, sex, race, age, teeth, hair, fingerprints, and so on. For the relatives and friends of the deceased, the body is that of an intimate or an associate; it is a body replete with meaning and personal memories, it is a subject body. While the police who conduct the process seek a positive identification, those asked to attend the mortuary to undertake the identification have exactly the opposite desire. They come with a fear of identification, dreading what they may find and hoping that they will not be able to make a positive identification. By identifying a body, family or close friends are being asked to claim that the corpse before them is not an object but a person, and, furthermore, a person whom they recognise.

'Jervis' notes a further difficulty of identification, one associated with asking relatives to undertake the task. 'It should be emphasised that caution is necessary since such inspection may be unpleasant and distressing for those concerned and they may pay too little attention and make an error' (Matthews and Foreman, 1993: 142). There are no statistics available to indicate the extent to which errors are made, but it could be argued that relatives who make errors are not simply 'paying too little attention'. Rather, they are responding to the dread of recognition and, in this process, are searching the corpse for alien or unfamiliar features. By searching for the strange characteristics, they may neglect or sub-rationally render the familiar invisible. In the materiality of the corpse, therefore, more than one social identity may be discerned.

The frequently prolonged impact of sudden death can complicate survivors' experience of bereavement, often because of the lack of time to prepare for death. Death is ordinarily viewed in a linear fashion, to be encountered at the end of the road of life. Sudden death is death out of time and out of place. It disrupts the biography; hence the need to construct a narrative which makes the death possible, indeed inevitable, for that person, in that place and at that time. Of particular significance for bereaved people is the fact that sudden death, together with the sudden loss of the body of the deceased as a source of sense-making, disrupts their own biographies, their own sense of self. The body of the deceased and the readings bereaved people take from the body, together with the expert readings presented to them during the inquest, aid them to move forward in their own lives – though often in directions they would never have chosen. They are enabled to take with them a clear perception of the deceased person and to fit an understanding of the death into their lives. The past needs to be reconstructed in such a way as to bring them to the present, and in so doing, to allow them to move on to the future. The reconstruction that occurs in the inquest can therefore be said to supplant the preparation for death.

The inquest

Given that relatives are rarely present when sudden death occurs, they too desire to reconstruct the event – the death of their loved one – in order to gain some understanding of their tragedy. Since they do not usually have access to expert reports or lay witness testimonies they must wait for the courtroom ritual to expose 'the facts' of the death, to hear witnesses depict the scene of death, and from these to be able to reconstruct the incident for themselves.

Lay witnesses might be called to shed light on the social circumstances surrounding death. They may be asked to comment on the character of the deceased or of any other person directly involved in the death. The discourse here centres on those present at the time of death, those first on the scene, or those with a contribution to make in terms of events leading up to the death; the deceased's state of mind, their relationship with others, their recent movements and actions, their apparent state of health, and so on. The purpose of lay testimony is to assist in spatially and temporally locating the person in that last phase of their life.

The expert reports make the internal condition of the body visible. The pathologist's report, for example, may detail the contents of the stomach; the amount of alcohol or drugs in the bloodstream. It may refer to the presence of old scars or wounds, or the marks left by medical interventions such as surgery. In more extreme cases, the professional testimonies may uncover information about a person's life that was hitherto unknown to relatives and friends. If this occurs, survivors may be forced to reassess their relationship with the deceased or even to reconstruct the dead person's identity, and as a consequence, aspects of their own self-identity. A sudden death brought about by pushing too far the boundaries of sexual excitement when experimenting with forms of sado-masochism may reveal information about sexual proclivities of which friends and family were unaware. A woman, for example, who 'thought she knew' her husband but had no knowledge of his sexual experiments, felt, in his death, that she did not really know him at all. She was forced to reconstruct his identity in the light of this new information – uncovered in death and known only through readings of the dead body. This demonstrates the point that despite the loss of agency as a property of the embodied self, empowerment persists at the site of the self. It is dynamically constructed and its inter-subjective nature is fore-grounded when others come to make sense of the biography of the deceased, produced in death. Alternatively, relatives and friends who knew the deceased may resist the courtroom reconstruction. In hearing the evidence they may be sceptical, unable, and unwilling to recognise the biography being constructed by the witnesses.

Foucault (1973; 1977) writes of the dominant institutional discourse in society and its capacity to construct the body. There are, however, sites of resistance to this dominant construction. The coroner's inquest can be one such site where bereaved people are busily constructing their own narratives and meanings of the dead body which may be made to stand in opposition to that of the professional readers. In this way, they do not necessarily reject the expert evidence but may employ it, often in fragmented forms, to piece together a lay or popular discourse on death. For sudden death is rarely a straightforward, uncomplicated event. Making sense of such death is often problematic. Scientific discourse, while describing the nature of the event, does not always extend the necessary insight demanded by the bereaved as the following case indicates.

When late one night a young man was seen to accidentally fall between the carriages of an underground train, momentarily stationed at a platform, the immediate response of fellow passengers and people on the platform was to attempt to signal to the driver that something was wrong. The driver, fearing a personal attack or other similar incident and aware that his technical equipment registered no alarm, pulled out of the station. The young man was crushed to death beneath the wheels of the train. At the inquest the pathologist was able to explain the nature of the man's injuries. He also noted that there were relatively high levels of alcohol in his blood. The police described the scene of the death and confirmed that the driver of the train had no alcohol or drugs in his bloodstream at the time of death. The railway inspector was able to point to the efficient working of health and safety procedures and the driver's union representative affirmed the professional manner in which the driver had conducted himself. The young man's companion that night, and other lay witnesses present on the platform, explained that they had seen the man fall and had tried to attract the attention of the driver. They also described the horror they experienced at seeing the train pull out of the station. The coroner's verdict was that the young man's death had been an 'accident'.

(Howarth, 1997)

For the family and friends this verdict was unacceptable and the testimonies of the experts were of little consequence to them. More than that, the expert evidence was considered by some family members to be irrelevant and in some ways offensive. The reason was that these professional accounts appeared to be defending the institutions and individuals who the family saw as blameworthy. Their testimonies were viewed either as merely descriptive or distanced explanations of the functioning of equipment or of the extent of the injuries the man had sustained in death. It did not matter that the driver had acted 'according to the book', 'anyone with any common sense' would conclude that he should not have started the train. In this particular case, for the intimates of the deceased, the popular discourse took precedence over the professional objective reports. Scientific and popular discourses often intersect and it is an aim of many coroners to ensure that each is pertinent to the other. Frequently, families may hear the expert testimonies and select fragments to fashion their own accounts of the death. Occasionally, as in the above account, there may be no meeting place for the two accounts.

The coroner has to take account of both scientific and popular discourses concerning the death and must use strategies to cut across and synthesize the two. Some coroners are expert intermediaries who see their role as mediating between the two discourses in order to produce an account of the deceased's life and death which is recognizable to all. Other coroners perceive their role as one which is more aligned to the scientific, objective and distanced explanations for the death, explanations which describe the death in ways which conform to the needs of the death certification process and the demands of public interest. According to the latter, the needs of the bereaved and their desire to make sense of their loss should play no part in translating the courtroom testimonies into a legal verdict.

There is, however, one verdict on sudden death which most coroners are at pains, if at all possible, to avoid passing: suicide. As the following chapter details, during the early modern period the body of the deceased needed to be presented in particular ways; the scene around the deathbed and the words of the dying person reported by witnesses using specific criteria to portray the death as a good one. In the case to be presented, a dying man was no longer able to speak and the testimonies of witnesses at the deathbed became particularly important. It was through their voices that the silent voice of the dead person was made audible. In the modern coroners' court, in the case of suicide, the biography of the deceased may be consciously written in a way which raises considerable doubt as to the nature of death; so much doubt, in fact, that the verdict becomes one of accident or misadventure. The actions, behaviour and voice of the dead person may not simply be silent but may be drowned out in the desire to recreate a good death – one which stigmatises neither the dead, nor the living.

In most other cases it is the production of a verdict, the official interpretation of the medical, legal and social discourse of the courtroom, which can result in a conflict or tension between the official purpose of the inquest and the expectations of the bereaved. The aftermath of the inquest for bereaved families is frequently characterised by bewilderment as they fail to understand the implications of the verdict and are left questioning the point of the inquiry. This can largely be attributed to the common expectation that 'something' will come out of the inquest. For many, this may take the form of an attribution of blame. For while the official purposes can be fulfilled by discovering the medical causes of death and by reaching a legal verdict, bereaved people need to construct a narrative of death which makes a sudden death possible – indeed, inexorable. In making the death inevitable, that is, in reconstructing the last moments or hours of the deceased's life, the question of causation is often linked with the notion of blame or responsibility. Vitebsky (1990) highlights a similar need in the inquests of the Sora people of central India. The interrogation of the dead, conducted by a shaman, entails learning details of which 'sonum' or 'spirit' caused the death. They ask:

> [w]hich sonum took you?...At the inquest you start putting together a picture of all the circumstances surrounding a person's death...And the verdict is summarized in the form of a certain explanation – it was this sonum, who did it for this reason.
>
> (Vitebsky, 1990: 40)

The logic of cause is compelling and it is interesting that both the Sora and the modern Western inquests interrogate the dead. For the Sora the shaman facilitates communion between the living and the dead; in Western systems it is the bodies of the dead that are explored and interrogated and found to contain causal knowledge. Non-Western cultures may look to causes such as witchcraft, malevolent ancestors, mistaken deeds. Western cultures ostensibly rely on the scientific explanations provided by the medical and the legal professions. Lay explanations, however, continue to set these objective accounts in a popular discourse that locates responsibility in more social terms, borrowing from the language of omen, fate, warnings, superstition, personal, social, institutional and corporate blame. For often, the language of science, which implies control, seems misleading and inadequate when employed to explain the event of sudden death. By definition, an event which is unexpected and uncontrolled has taken place. While scientific discourse may retrospectively furnish an objective explanation for the event and propose ways in which the fatality might be avoided in the future, it has nothing to offer the lay person seeking to comprehend why that particular death was not avoided on this occasion. Here we find a parallel with material on witchcraft among the Azande where common sense and magical explanations complement rather than compete with one another. Though there is a common-sense acknowledgement that the material world can indeed collapse around one – quite literally, when granaries on stilts keel over – there remains the more fateful question of why such an event should take place 'here' and 'now' (Evans-Pritchard, 1937).

Conclusion

Having detailed knowledge of the end of a person's life gives the biographer the power to recreate, or indeed, to create a biographical account that matches or fits the final acts of life. As McCann argues in his work on biography, reading a life can destroy and simultane-ously create our image of the subject (1991: 329). There are parallels here between the coroner's inquest, the work of literary biographers and the accounts of witnesses presented during early modern testamentary disputes. This chapter has shown that, as a material object, the body in death becomes a source of information, its surveillance and the readings taken from the corpse generating narrative reconstructions of a former life. The chapter which follows details a similar process of retrospective interrogation of the dying body. In both cases we see how readings at the site of the dying and dead body lead back to the life that has been lost, creating particular images or biographies of that person. In contemporary society there is an assumption that life is encoded in death, the truth of which can be discovered from internal examinations of the body. From both internal and external examinations of the body, and expert and lay interpretations of its meanings, the 'facts' of death are discursively constructed within the coroner's court. Though silent and inert, the dead body retains agency and continues to be integral to the production and experience of the social reality of sudden death. Constructed rather than self-constructing, an identity is imposed on the deceased, an identity formulated from readings of the body and the nature of death. As data presented here indicate, that identity can contradict previous identities if the body reveals secrets about the nature of an individual's life formerly unknown.

Chapter 6

Narratives of the body II
The Church court[1]

This chapter complements the previous chapter's focus on reading the dying and dead body with an examination of witnesses' accounts which were produced for early modern court cases where a will was in dispute. Central to discussion here is the spoken and written word and its social and cultural significance in the production of social identity during the dying process. Bronfen and Goodwin focus on the relationship between the deceased and testamentary texts, highlighting the social agency of the dead as mediated through writing practices. They move on to probe to the nature and authority of the 'voice' which the will might provide for the corpse:

> [t]o give a voice to the corpse, to represent the body, is in a sense to return it to life: the voice represents not so much the dead as the once living, juxtaposed with the needs of the yet living.
>
> (Bronfen and Goodwin, 1993: 7)

> Does the testamentary will represent the corpse? What kind of voice does the body have in the text, the linguistic traces, it leaves behind? Does the signature represent the corpse? If so, then it surely also represents a good deal more: the corpse come back to life, so to speak, as a powerful social force.
>
> (ibid.: 6)

In the context of early modern death rituals, writing and the production of texts were intimately tied to embodied experience: codes of conduct, gestures and the condition of the body all impinged upon the writing of the will. It could be argued that the body itself formed a text, exhibiting signs which were interpreted by deathbed attendants. To ensure the effective writing of the will, the dying body was required to communicate unambiguous messages: clear speech and orderly, ritualised gestures would secure the effective writing of will. Witnesses' retrospective descriptions of the condition of the body were also crucial in guaranteeing the authenticity of the will in that the body was seen to express the genuine will. In the case study presented within this chapter we examine the accounts of a dying body which failed to meet the social expectations of the 'good death'. Such a dying body was troubling in its lack of the necessary social expressivity and we find witnesses attempting, in court, to assign meaning and provide explanation. In so doing, witnesses traced the possible intentions of the deceased, piecing together fragments of life history to make sense of a death and to guide the effective execution of the will.

Prioritising the word

Our analysis here takes as its starting point the relationships between the dying body and the production of texts, and in particular the writing and reading practices conducted at the deathbed in early modern England. As one of the key phases of transition in the life course, the process of dying was ritualised to the extent that preparations for the point of death were conducted sometimes over a number of years. The notion that 'life was death and death was life' underpinned many sixteenth- and seventeenth century sermons (Cressy, 1997: 382). For instance Cressy quotes one sermon from 1595, '[f]or when we are born we are mortal, but when we are dead we are immortal. And we are alive in the womb to die in the world, but we are dead in the grave to live in heaven' (ibid.: 384). Souls were believed to depart bodies at death, earthly bodies would then decay but those of the faithful would be reunited with the soul in heaven (ibid.: 384–385). Llewellyn also highlights the perceived continuities between life and death during this period, and with regard to conceptions of the dead body he notes its division into two 'aspects': 'The first, the social body after death, is sustained in our memories by artefacts...; the second, the natural body after death is lifeless, alien and used up' (1991: 9). While Llewellyn explores the visual images and material objects associated with death, we complement this approach with an examination of textual representations linked to the dying body and death. In the Church court records which document will making practices, we find descriptions of social relationships and practices which reinforce continuities between the living and the dead. Through will making and the legal processes that surrounded the contestation of wills, narratives encompassing aspects of the life history of the deceased were produced. As already demonstrated in the previous chapter, a similar retrospective reconstruction of life histories centring upon the dead body takes place in contemporary Western legal settings, such as the coroner's court. With reference to the early modern period, we here explore lay and legal discourses as they related to the dying body and the preservation of the social agency of the deceased. Through a detailed case study, the method which has been used throughout the book, we discover that the writing of the will, as well as aspects of Church court writing practices, were intimately related to the condition of the dying body and the construction of the social identity of the deceased. First, however, we contextualise the case study in relation to early modern death rituals and deathbed practices, examining gender relations, notions of bodily conduct, and perceptions of the dying body.

In relation to sociological debates about the historical roots of individualism, Mellor and Shilling point to the emergence of, what they term, 'Protestant modern bodies'. They identify three key aspects of the protestant reformation with regard to concepts of the body:

> First,...in prioritising cognitive belief and thought as routes to knowledge, Protestantism made linguistic symbols and narratives, (which could be thought with, spoken and read) a central source of peoples self-identity. Second, the Protestant flesh was something which had to be made subordinate to these (religiously justifiable) narratives; the body had, in other words to be controlled by the mind. Third, the ultimate inability of these narratives fully to control human emotions and passions helps us understand the enormous degree of anxiety stimulated in Protestants over those sinful aspects of their bodily selves (and the bodies of others) which threatened to become grotesque and out of control.
>
> (Mellor and Shilling, 1997: 42)

This emphasis on the control of the flesh and the prioritising of the word, is evidenced in the circulation of conduct and advice books which provided guidance on bodily comportment and gesture, while linking these to issues of social morality and spirituality.

These texts were related to the social and cultural emphasis on manners from the sixteenth century onwards and were written for pedagogical purposes to instruct in appropriate bodily etiquette. They were based on the assumption that

> physical signs – gestures, mimicry, postures – express a person's inner state in an intelligible fashion, revealing the disposition of the soul.... [e]very physical movement and gesture lends itself to similar interpretation, as does clothing. Gestures are signs and as such can be organised into a language, interpreted and read as moral, psychological and social markers. By such signs even the most intimate secrets are betrayed.
>
> (Revel, 1989, 169–170)

To establish a common code of manners, 'social transparency' was necessary such that gestures or speeches which were likely to cause confusion with regard to their meanings became problematic (ibid.: 171). The dying body and the socially disorderly body as sources of 'opaque' or confusing social signs and messages are examined later in this chapter.

Of particular relevance here is the dissemination of texts relating to conduct during the dying process and also in the sphere of sexuality. Both of these areas of bodily conduct, associated with different stages of the life cycle, were subject to discipline and control through conduct literature as well as the legal practices of local Church courts. The socially approved 'good death', during which 'speech, emotions and actions' were controlled, was guided by codes of conduct to be observed at the deathbed. 'Anxieties were to be calmed, and bodies stilled, through the reading and interpreting of texts' (Mellor and Shilling, 1997: 120). Cressy notes the significance of the *ars moriendi* (art of dying) in the later sixteenth and early seventeenth centuries.

> Ideally, according to Christian council, the deathbed would be attended by ministers and friends, neighbours and kin, who would share godly comfort and bear witness to a satisfactory passing. If blessed by God, the fortunate Christian would be fully articulate to the end.... Children as well as adults were watched for signs of fortitude and grace, and their silences as well as utterances were weighed for spiritual significance.
>
> (Cressy, 1997: 309)

Guidance on the good death was provided in Christian biographies, and diaries contain reflections on deathbed practices (ibid.: 392). The ritualised performance of will making, the settlement of the estate and the confirmation of relationships between family and friends ensured that these codes of conduct were communicated and reinforced through social practice (Hallam, 1996).

In a similar way the excesses of sexuality were addressed through advice books and marriage manuals. As Jones notes, the proliferation of practical conduct books in the sixteenth century meant that 'women were consistently the objects of scrutiny and the targets of complex prescriptions for proper behaviour' (1987: 39). Jones argues further that:

> the most widely disseminated feminine ideal was the confinement of the bourgeois daughter and wife to private domesticity in the households of city merchants, professional men and, in England, protestant fathers and husbands. The court lady was required to speak; the bourgeois wife enjoined to silence.
>
> (1987: 40)

Emphasis was placed upon women's effective performance of household duties, as well as the preservation of the purity of their bodies and the regulation of their speech.

> The good wife was constructed as the woman who stays in doors, guarding her chastity as she guards the other property of her husband. As her body is locked within the walls of the house, her tongue is locked in her mouth.
>
> (ibid.: 52)

Ideas regarding the control of the female body formed significant aspects of gender ideologies which constructed hierarchical relationships between men and women. Men's authority, to a certain extent, rested upon representations of the female body as prone to sexual temptations, disorderly and in need of control (Fletcher, 1995). Women were represented as a source of sin and, indeed, death (see Chapter 2). However, cultural representations of women within the site of death were complex in that they encompassed conflicting images of, on the one hand, the value and necessity of women's work at the deathbed and, on the other, the female physical form as a cause of disorder and death (see Hallam, 1997a).

With its emphasis on perceptions of the dying body, this chapter traces some of these complexities.

While social historians of the early modern period have analysed extended rituals after the point of death, focusing upon public funerals, little attention has been paid to the embodied aspects of deathbed ritual and the management of the dying body in this context. Bodily transformations and the accompanying changes in social relations which occur throughout the life course, have been conceptualised primarily in terms of rites of passage which are seen to ease and contain the tensions invoked by these changes. Rites of passage function to symbolically mark bodily changes and shifts in social identity, but they have been analysed in terms of their functions in the maintenance of established social and power structures. From this perspective, the threat of various changes at physical and social levels and their capacity to disrupt social relations are contained by the efforts made during ritual to achieve symbolic resolution and closure. Huntington and Metcalf (1979) analyse these issues in relation to mortuary rituals. They suggest that the ambiguities in social relations that death presents are, to a certain extent, resolved and organised during rites of passage. They describe a variety of rites, all of which are underpinned by a similar structure. With reference to the Bara of Madagascar they argue that:

> one can view the whole funeral sequence as a single rite of passage, seeing the original burial as a rite of separation, the gathering as a period of liminality, and the reburial as the ceremony of reintegration. It is a question of how wide a per-spective one takes. There are transitions within transitions within transitions.
>
> (ibid.: 118)

They argue that it is possible to describe the complexity of emotions, ritual actions and beliefs associated with death, in various cultures, within the 'universal rite of passage schema' (ibid.: 99). While historians have analysed death in the context of religious and social change, there has remained an emphasis upon dying and death as a rite of passage structured in the manner suggested by Huntington and Metcalf. Beaver has commented upon recent historical studies arguing that most of these have tended to approach death through demography rather than the 'social experience of death' (Beaver, 1992: 390). He argues that although there has been a move away from the general study of Western attitudes to death, as exemplified in Ariès's work, towards an appreciation of the significance of social context, still there had been a failure to 'explicate the symbolism and social content of mortuary customs' (ibid.: 392). Acknowledging the importance of work which has identified the implications of Reformation for the rituals surrounding death, as in Houlbrooke's analysis of death within the family (Houlbrooke, 1989: 25–42), Beaver nevertheless proposes that a closer analysis of death ritual and symbolism at the local level is required. He recognises that members of different social groups will have a different experience of death, but argues for a unity of structure in death ritual.

> In the early modern mortuary system, the preparation of a will, the funeral procession, the burial and the construction of a memorial accomplished distinct symbolic tasks in the process of movement from the hierarchic social order of the visible world to the egalitarian social order of the Christian afterlife. These symbolic elements of the mortuary process commemorated and closed the position of the dying person in the everyday life of local society.
>
> (Beaver, 1992: 418)

Such studies continue to stress the significance of life crisis ritual in the maintenance of 'social order' predicated upon the maintenance of boundaries between social groups and categories. The threats that death represents for social and symbolic structures are recognised but it is argued that these rituals were largely successful in containing these. The functional capacity of death ritual is also emphasised by Cressy in his study of the funerals of Essex gentry in the late sixteenth century. He argues that these rituals 'affirmed the local social hierarchy which the parish gentry dominated' (Cressy 1989: 99–119). From this perspective the crises which emerged during the process of dying were contained by rituals which ultimately reinforced established social and power relations.

The historical perspectives outlined above are heavily influenced by earlier anthropological work which examined ritual as clearly defined, simple linear sequences of action with distinct spatial and temporal boundaries organised into a tripartite structure (Van Gennep, [1909] 1960; Huntington and Metcalf, 1979). However, recent studies of ritual performance signal a departure from this approach. Representing ritual from a single perspective is problematic in that it does not acknowledge the diversity of embodied experiences and interpretations that are possible within any given ritual context. Parkin argues that 'ritual is held to privilege action; but it is an action that can only be understood as bodily movement towards or positioning with respect to other bodily movements and positions' (1992: 12). In other words, the relationships between different embodied orientations are key aspects of ritual practice. Furthermore, bodily 'movement, directionality, and positioning' are likely to be contested as 'rivals compete to control the conduct of rituals in order to legitimate leadership roles' (ibid.: 12–13). In addition to this emphasis on bodily conduct, we also note anthropological approaches which question the stability of boundaries which separate ritual from routine social action (for example, Rosaldo, 1989). Serematakis argues that:

> a treatment of mourning rituals which acknowledges the problematic nature of discrete beginnings and endings also assumes that there is never a full restoration of social stability; that death, its representation, its discourses, and its performative elaboration can haunt society and become an essential collective metaphor of social experience beyond the margins of ceremonial performance.
>
> (1991: 48)

Following these anthropological insights into the instability of boundaries and the centrality of the body, we here explore perceptions of the dying body as well as the continued social presence of the departed, as evidenced in the ritualised writing surrounding the making and execution of wills. The experience and effects of the early modern dying process were not confined to the immediate death event. Dying was discussed, remembered and referred to in various social contexts and over considerable periods of time.

It is, therefore, important to acknowledge the written and spoken word as part of the social and cultural processes which impinged upon death and its meanings. The following discussion provides a wider social and cultural context for the case study, focusing on will making, the textual aspects of this process, and the ritualised dimensions of the deathbed which shaped perceptions of the dying body.

Witnessing and recollecting death

During the late sixteenth and early seventeenth centuries the Church courts were responsible for the management of testamentary business. The analysis here is based on witnesses' accounts from the Church courts in Canterbury between 1580 and 1640 (Hallam, 1994). These form detailed descriptions, recorded in court during the proceedings of legal action taken when wills were disputed. Where the contents of the will were not seen accurately to reflect the deceased's wishes or when the executors had not performed their duties, legal action might be sought (Houlbrooke, 1979). Once the legal process had begun, the focus of the investigations tended to widen and encompass a range of issues dealing with the relationships and actions of the dying person. Witnesses brought into court to provide evidence described various stages and different aspects of the will making process, from the initial stages of will making through to the deathbed and on to arrangements made after the testator's death. Although some wills, especially those of high status men in Canterbury, were begun well in advance of any sickness, witnesses provided detailed descriptions of the deathbed as it was regarded as the most important site for confirming the last wishes of the person. Such accounts form an important source of information regarding the encounters which took place during the hours, days, months and, in some cases, years before the moment of death. They also provide a rich source for the analysis of perceptions of the body, social relations and ritual practices during the dying process. The relationships between the embodied process of dying, witnesses' observations of this process and the written representation of the witnesses' verbal account of the process, in the form of the deposition, are complex. An acknowledgement of this complexity involves the identification of the deposition document as a text shaped by a range of legal as well as social and cultural practices emerging over time. From this perspective the deposition document stands as a constructed representation, subject to the forces and tensions of gender and power relations within and beyond the ecclesiastical courts. When the officials of the courts called a witness to give an account of what they had seen of the deceased during the period before death they activated a process of recollection and verbal description.

The resulting spoken accounts were then translated into written documents as part of the record keeping of court officials. Officials' interests were mainly directed towards the resolution of dispute and to this end witnesses were encouraged to provide the court with an honest account of the deceased's last wishes and state of mind as well as assurance that the appropriate conduct had been observed around the deathbed (Houlbrooke, 1979). This tended to result in accounts which represented dying as a series of encounters concerned with the distribution of property through will making.

The writing of the will document, the witnessing and final confirmation of the last will, figured as significant moments during the time before death. Witnesses' descriptions of dying were, therefore, constructed within the legal discourse of the courts and this tended to push witnesses' accounts in particular directions. The image of the deathbed, the site of the dying body, was commonly located at the centre of witnesses' accounts acting as a focus for narratives concerned with the daily routines of the dying. The deathbed assumed particular significance as an organising feature of depositions. Witnesses repeatedly referred to this site when describing the relations and encounters between the dying and their family and friends. In instances where the disputed contents of a will gave rise to legal action there were at least two phases of textual production which were part of the process of dying. These were the writing of the will document and the record making which accompanied the legal resolution of the will dispute. Both phases of textual production involved ritualised action which was, for the most part, organised and performed by men working as officials and professionals in the church and city. In their capacity as producers of legal documentation men made important contributions towards the management of the dying process. This points towards a gendered division of labour which worked to exclude women's access to a form of textual production which was also an important means of representing social relations. As men exercised authority over will making and the legal practices which tended to structure witnesses' perceptions and accounts of dying, it might be argued that the meanings and values attributed to deathbed practices were products of a gendered hierarchy which privileged men and continued to reproduce gender inequalities. However, the contents of witnesses' accounts were also subject to various pressures and tensions which came into play well before the legal procedures had begun. Thus deposition texts cannot be regarded as products constructed exclusively by (male) official requirements. Witnesses brought their own experiences and interpretations to bear when speaking in court. The narrative focus upon the deathbed was also a result of personal and emotional investment. It represented a phase of personal and social adjustment to imminent loss.

Although families and friends were obliged to recognise and follow officially sanctioned procedures at the deathbed they also brought their own gestures and interpretations into the process. These constituted another set of gendered meanings which might intersect with those generated by legal practice but, equally, might not engage with it directly. The deathbed formed a site where an intensity of personal, moral and legal interests gathered and where the heightened interplay of sentiment and ritualised action ensured that it figured strongly in recollections of dying. A description of this diversity of interest and action within the space of the deathbed opens the possibility for an analysis of the ways women contributed to its management. In addition, it indicates some of the interventions women made in the cultural production and maintenance of the meanings surrounding death.

Gender, signs and tokens

Witnesses' descriptions of death beds often included details regarding the physical condition of the dying person and indicate the perceived importance of certain embodied forms of communication. The indications that death was approaching were usually communicated by the suffering person to women within the household. Their receptivity towards the signs of death was highlighted in several witnesses' accounts (C.C.A.L., MSS., DCb. X.11.1, f.155, 157, October 1587). The witnessing by women of these 'statements' formed an important part in the recognition that death was near. Women's presence and support were important aspects of the encounters when the proximity of death was announced. They therefore contributed towards a reflexive process whereby the sick verbally articulated their entry into the final life phase.

Women were also called upon to search for and interpret 'tokens' of the inner condition which were visibly manifested on the surface of the physical body and through gestures during the dying process. The roles of 'looker', 'nurse', 'attendant' or constant observer of the deathbed were particularly important as they actively engaged women in an interpretative process which mediated the deathbed and wider social relations. This was a labour which rested upon interpretative skill and a sensitivity of perception regarding the dynamics between personal, social and spiritual domains activated at times of crisis. Signs and tokens were received by observers as indications of the mental, spiritual and physical condition of the dying person. The face and hands were seen as especially expressive of the inner self and they were exposed to intensive observation and visual interrogation at the deathbed. Tokens which emerged upon the body or through gesture indicated a fading or a weakening of communication with the living. As the face and hands lost their animation and expressive vigour, they signalled a distancing from the immediate social environment. Women in the position of lookers were the primary mediators between the dying person and their close family and friends.

The deathbed was a space which developed a rich visual and aural texture, where each word and gesture became meaningful in physical, social and spiritual terms. Women would often decipher these signs and tokens in 'word' and 'deed', in 'expression' or 'gesture' (see Chapter 10 on women reading bodily signs). This was not an activity which was expected of and performed exclusively by women, as doctors and ministers were also concerned with the bodily indications of physical and spiritual health. But women did share daily routines in households and neighbourhoods with those they attended and this provided access to the intimate knowledge upon which women's readings of such signs were based. Women's domestic relationships, established well before the onset of dying, afforded them special access to the intentions displayed at deathbed. In addition, women's longer-term commitment at the deathbed was recognised as important when it came to interrogating any ambiguity surrounding the intentions of the deceased. Women were trusted observers of the dying and 'honest' women's interpretations of tokens during life crises carried legal weight. Their speeches were well received, by lay persons and church officials alike, as reliable representations.

While the dying body defined the main symbolic arena with which women were concerned, men were more centrally involved in the practices surrounding the will document. There was a continuity between these two arenas as will making was best performed when the dying person was in an orderly, settled condition. Women attendants would labour to comfort the dying person so they remained in a state acceptable to will makers. Women acted as mediators between the dying person and male specialists positioned to facilitate the confirmation of the dying person's last wishes. This was most explicit when wives called their male kin to the deathbed to ensure that the will was completed (C.C.A.L., MSS., DCb PRC39/37, f.195, 198, August 1626). A body 'at ease' and a quiet and settled mind was required so that orderly words could be spoken and then written into an acceptable document (C.C.A.L., MSS., DCb X.11.14, f.108, 113, April 1623). Noise and uninhibited actions, angry or idle speech and disorderly gestures could all disrupt will making. Women's efforts to settle and encourage testators in preparation for the declaration of their last wishes were often described by witnesses (C.C.A.L., MSS., DCb PRC39/44, f.260, 267, June 1636).

Women's informed readings of the signs of death were valuable in that they initiated a process of preparation essential for a 'good death' (Beier, 1989). Once a person was perceived to be beyond recovery, a series of obligations and expectations were brought into play. A person must be prepared for death and their spiritual condition attended to; their final wishes regarding their material possessions should be confirmed; and their relationships with family, kin, friends and neighbours should be acknowledged. Dying was expected to take the form of a gradual process which allowed enough time for social and spiritual adjustment, combined with the orderly settlement of the final will. Sudden death, or unanticipated death was problematic and distressing. The gender divisions which emerged during different phases of the dying process did not always involve antagonism or conflict as the different gender groups might work with a degree of co-operation towards a 'good death'.

Despite this continuity between the contributions of women and men there was a distinct boundary which marked the distancing and sometimes the exclusion of women from will making practices. This boundary was invoked in a variety of ways, depending upon several factors, including wealth and status. The exclusion of women was most clearly emphasised when the testator was a man of considerable wealth and high status and in situations where tensions had developed between the testator and his wife (C.C.A.L., MSS., DCb PRC39/35, f.274–275, March 1621; DCb PRC39/47, f.54, 74–75, November 1637). Women found less resistance towards their involvement when the testator was a woman and when the will was spoken. Men from family, kin and professional groups reserved control over the writing, amending, reading and ritualised confirmation of the will. It was perceived to be a ritual object rather than a 'transparent' document which functioned merely to hold information about the transfer of property. The physical appearance of the document, with its marks and seals was as significant as the content of the written text. Furthermore, the document was constructed and activated through a series of ritualised practices which involved speech, gesture and the giving of tokens, all of which became imbued with emotional, social and spiritual meanings. Wills were written in draft and then 'fayre' copies suggesting that a special style of writing was reserved for the final document. Seal rings worn on the hand, and the seals they imprinted, carried the sign of the testator and helped in identifying the document as valid. They also served as symbolic confirmation of relationships between men (C.C.A.L., MSS., DCb PRC39/32, f.80,118, 123, 211–213, June 1614; DCb PRC39/34, f.68–73, September 1618).

The representations produced throughout the will making process foregrounded issues of secrecy, exclusion and enclosure. These issues were intimately related to gender and power relations and were often present within the repeated and complex representation of the will document itself, with its attendant seals, boxes and locks. The spatial location of this document was also reinforced when men engaged in private and secret conference over wills. The study formed the most secluded place for such exchanges. This seclusion was a sign of control and authority and only a select few within the city could boast access to a space which was so effectively removed from public view (C.C.A.L., MSS., DCb PRC39/46, f.36–37, 40–41, October 1634).

Silent and disorderly bodies: a case study

As noted above, during the sixteenth and seventeenth centuries there was a growing concern with regard to bodily comportment which was increasingly subject to social and legal scrutiny. Through this case study, we examine the perceived interdependence of the dying body and the disorderly conduct of a woman, as represented by Church court witnesses during an early modern will dispute. The written documents generated during this legal case account for one man's physical, emotional and moral decline before death in relation to his daughter's domestic transgressions. His entry into a

phase of 'silence' and 'senselessness' became particularly problematic in a context where the final wishes of the dying were
confirmed through the spoken word. We explore the contested
meanings which were attributed by witnesses to the distressed,
inarticulate and immobile body. The stories which emerged to
explain this physical state cohere around the disorderly conduct of
a woman – the dying man's daughter – which was perceived to
have destabilised the household.

What follows is the story of one man's sudden death and the
attempts by those who knew him to make sense of this death in the
context of the legal process, witnesses went to court to provide
'evidence' which would lead to the resolution of the will dispute.
They described various relationships, emotional attachments and
intentions which they saw as evident from the actions of the
deceased before his death. The will was contested mainly because
neither a 'good' death', nor the expected codes of orderly conduct,
gesture and speech, were achieved in this case. Instead, the
witnesses described the dying man's physical condition as one
which was deeply troubling and, indeed, linked to the destabilised
household relationships and tensions that surrounded him. At the
centre of this case lie descriptions of a dying body which was
'silent' and unable to communicate. In a sense, he was seen as
socially dead, in that he was unable to participate in the social
interactions which would have maintained his position within a
network of social and personal relationships. The dying man's lack
of direct social agency, during the point at which he was expected
to express his will, led to the production of retrospective narratives
relating to his life which would recover this agency.

Stephen Brett was resident in Canterbury before he died and
during the legal case, fourteen witnesses mainly from the same city
but also from Biddenden, Sandwich, Norborne and Portsmouth
went to court in June 1634 to provide evidence (C.C.A.L, MSS,
DCb/PRC 39/45, fo. 65, 71, 85, 90, 109–112, 116). Witnesses' accounts
centre upon the distressing physical condition of Stephen Brett in
the hours before his death. Laurence Omer of St George's parish
had

> heard that the satterday in the night time the evening next
> befor his death having received great hurt by a fall he then had
> did grow soe extraordinary sick and ill that ther with he was

bereft of his sences memory and understanding and from that
time not perceived by any one to speake.

[Brett, 1634]

With the loss of 'senses, memory and understanding' as well as his
capacity to speak Brett had entered into a problematic bodily state
which triggered various responses form various neighbours, friends
and professionals. William Berry, a gentleman with whom Brett was
living, described the night before Brett died. Brett had 'receaved a
hurt by a fall' and afterwards

> was set in a chaire by the fireside where…[Berry] coming to
> him and finding him asleep which he conceved proceeded from
> his excessive drinking went to bedd and left him there suppos-
> ing he would be better the next morning and gave his mayd a
> chardge to sitt by him and look unto him all that night and the
> next day this deponent arising early…came to him againe and
> finding him rather worse then better went to one of his neigh-
> bours and asked his opinion what he were best to doe unto him
> and from him went to Mr Foxe a churgeon and brought him
> along with him to….[Brett] to surch what hurt he had received
> that soe he might apply or use his best skill in helping him and
> after again went to Mr Randolph dr of Physick and acquainted
> him in what condicion…[he] then was and had binn all night
> before and the concieved occasion whence his illness proceeded
> who therupon wished this respondent to let him alone a while
> longer saying that if he should goe unto him in the day time
> people would take notice ther of and so he said …[Brett's] good
> name or credit might be called in question but told this re-
> spondent that if he did not suddenly recover or grow better he
> would come unto him if he had notice therof and afterwards
> before his death being sent unto did come.

The morning after the 'fall' Berry had taken Brett from the fireside
into a chamber upstairs Brett 'being unable to go himself'. He was
undressed and helped into bed. Brett was then accompanied by Mr
Fox, the surgeon, but he died soon afterwards.

The witnesses' accounts of this troubling death moved into
descriptions which accounted for it in a variety of ways, all of which
would have implications for the distribution of the deceased's estate.
It was Easter day and Brett was known to have been drinking all

day in a tavern until the evening before he died. So there were suspicions that he was drunk although, as Omer deposed, Brett was 'reputed a sober man'. Thomas Coleman of St George, a beer brewer, confirmed that the night before Brett died when he returned home from the tavern he was 'much neglected and left comfortlesse'. This neglect was, to a certain extent, blamed upon Brett's servant Elizabeth Budd and Brett's own daughter, Thomasina Netter. Coleman had heard that 'when he [Brett] last kept house he was much troubled with his maid servant' and was 'constrained to go to markett and buy his provision himself for a quarter of a year'. Brett had also claimed that the 'discurtesies and unkindness which he received from his daughter were the only causes that mad him leave of housekeeping and betake himself to sojourning'. Edmund Randolph, a doctor of St Margaret's parish, had information to add in this respect. He had heard Brett say that it was the carelessness and negligence of servants and 'not any dislike he took against his daughter was the only cause that made him give over housekeeping and betake himself to sojourning'. Witnesses therefore saw women's neglect of domestic duties as a force which drove Stephen Brett to move from his house and into lodgings.

William Berry, a gentleman living in St George, provided a detailed account of Stephen Brett's past family relations, illness and emotional condition. A year before Brett's death he had 'kept house' with his widowed daughter and he had been distressed by her conduct. He had complained many times to Berry about

[the] demeanuries gestures and carriage of his daughter towards him at which he much grieved and seemed to be very much discontented and would often protest that such her unkind and discurteous carriage towards him would make him leave off housekeeping and betake himself againe to sojourning.

Brett had also been 'troubled and molested' by his daughter's husband's debts before the husband died. Thomas Brett, brother of the deceased, represented the behaviour of Stephen Brett's daughter as a contributory factor in Brett's illness and death. Thomas Brett deposed that his brother came to visit him in London or elsewhere once a year and

at the least of those times always complained of the disobedience of and unquietnes of Thomazine Netter his daughter and especially toward his latter time that he was weary of his life in respect of her unquiet carriage towards him because she did continually thwart him and crosse him in all things he did or undertooke and was not soe careful of him as he expected she should have been and that he was fearful that she would undoe her children by her negligence and carelesnes in their education.

Brett also told his brother that he intended to leave housekeeping 'which he said proceeded all from the unquietness and disrespect he received by living with his daughter the which he expressed with tears in his eyes'.

These discussions, according to Thomas Brett, took place about a year before Brett died. The emotional distress which was seen to arise out of his disapproval of Thomazine Netter's behaviour was perceived to have driven him to abandon his house and 'sojourne' at William Berry's house. Brett also observed that Stephen Brett's 'love and affection became alienated and estranged to his said daughter and her children'. Given the affection he had formerly held for Brett Netter, his grandson, this separation would have been emotionally distressing. Thomas Brett added that

> the disobedience of Thomazine Netter was the only cause that forced...[Brett] to sojourne abroad...if he had continued quietly at home he might have lived longer and so by that means she was a remote cause of...[Brett's] unhappie and untimely death the more imediate cause of the suddanness of...[his] death was by reason of the fall or hurt he tooke when he came from the taverne and his being neglected afterwards.

As an 'intimate and familiar acquaintance', William Berry saw that Stephen Brett did

> very intirely and affectionately love and affect Brett Netter his daughters sonne and seemed to be much delighted with his actions speech and gestures and gave him money to buy him paper to make pictures on and would shew those pictures to this respondent [Berry] and others of his acquaintance and say they were pictures of his boy Brett Netters making.

Berry perceived that Brett's 'affection was such and soe great unto Brett Netter that if he had lived he would ther after have brought up Brett Netter at the university or Inns of Court'. Brett also appeared to have intended to bequeath his estate to his grandson as he had taken the boy out to see his land in various parts of Kent and on his return, Brett had told his friends about the visits. The witnesses in this case provided accounts of Stephen Brett's emotional condition during the year before he died. Although he appeared 'healthy' to some, he also displayed unhappiness.

While living with his widowed daughter and her children he had become discontented and disapproved of her behaviour. Thomazine Netter was said to be disobedient, unquiet and lacking in care. Her behaviour had 'alienated' her father's 'love and affection' and it was feared that her 'negligence and carelesness' would 'undoe' her children. She was perceived to be a disorderly woman who had driven her father from his home. Brett's daughter was seen to be 'unquiet' and neglectful of familial and domestic duties. This conduct, especially in the absence of her deceased husband, ran counter to expected codes of conduct for women. The distress involved in this disruption was then linked, in the accounts, to Brett's death. Brett was perceived to be 'grieved' and 'discontented' during the year before his death and when this was combined with drinking 'to excess' and a 'fall' Brett became 'extraordinary sick and ill that ther with he was bereft of his sences memory and understanding'.

Thus, the legal process involved in the will dispute provided a forum in which narratives of the emotions, relationships and intentions of the deceased were reconstructed. The death had been sudden and unexpected, leaving no time to prepare a 'good death'. A written will, with all of its symbolic and social ramifications had not been completed, leaving intentions with regard to the distribution of the estate unclear. In the context of disrupted family relationships, in which particular gendered roles (especially those expected of women) had not been fulfilled, we find accounts of a particularly distressing death.

The dying body, in this case, was interpreted through a matrix of disharmonious relationships. Ideally, at the deathbed, the dying person was expected to engage in embodied forms of communication which would clarify intentions and confirm the social significance of familial relationships. In this case, the dying man was unable to express himself within this language. As a result a legal testamentary process was initiated and this gave rise to the production of narratives centring on the dying body. Accounts of the problematic condition of this dying body linked it to the disruptive actions of the deceased's daughter. As discussed above, social concerns regarding the conduct of women, and their embodied nature, came into play to provide a framework for the interpretation of a disorderly death. The implications of this process of narration are twofold. They reinforced particular cultural stereotypes regarding the disorderly capacities of women, linking them into a pattern of causation which began with female disobedience and ended in the death of a man. They were also part of a process of memory making which was regarded as necessary in the settlement of an estate, but which also ensured the continued social agency of the deceased.

Conclusions

Like the sudden deaths which the coroner judges it necessary to investigate, deaths of the kind described above fail to map on to conceptions of the 'good' death. They resist the classifactory frameworks through which a degree of control is exercised over the unpredictability and disorder which death can be felt to represent. In the wealth of detail which is drawn upon in the construction of a retrospective 'biography' of those who, in some form, have died a 'bad' death, we gain some measure of the intensity with which the need to make sense of a death can be felt. In both these case studies it becomes apparent that interpretations of physical changes within the body which lead to death are profoundly cultural, reflecting as they do the key social, moral and legal issues of their day. And, as emphasised throughout, these interpretations frequently reflect a process of negotiation if not contestation between experts and lay people, women and men. They should not be read as reflections of any kind of secure consensus.

Note

[1] Part of this chapter was published in Hallam, E. (1996), 'Turning the hourglass: gender relations at the deathbed in early modern Canterbury'. *Mortality*, 1 (1) 61–82. The present version has been revised and updated.

Chapter 7

Socialising the body

While social anthropologists have long acknowledged the importance of the dead body, recording insights into cultural aspects of its dress, decoration and preparation for disposal (see for example, Bloch, 1994: 145–146), sociologists have tended to restrict their gaze to the living body. Indeed, as noted earlier, this is a relatively recent area of sociological enquiry. None the less it has already established the cultural significance of the living body as a source of well-being, with the body's demeanour being identified as a critical key to personhood. For medical sociologists in particular, analyses of bodily behaviour and meanings have produced insights into how people perceive their bodies and the effect of bodily transformation on their sense of well-being and self-identity (Kleinman, 1988). When we report illness to our doctors they examine the body and read it for signs of malaise and disease (Helman, 1990). Indeed, we scrutinise our own bodies and the signs of health or illness which we find affect the way we feel and the confidence with which we face the world (Radley, 1994). The media and health promotion literature are replete with images of the beautiful, young, sexual, fit, muscular, slim bodies to which we are all invited to aspire (Lupton, 1996). Inextricably linked with these images is the growth in mass consumerism and the expansion, since the mid-century, of consumer products to aid and encourage us in our attempts to achieve the perfect body (Featherstone, 1991).

But if the body is a source of pleasure, health, beauty and youth, it is also potentially dangerous and threatening as a site of contamination, disease and disorder (Douglas, 1966; Howarth, 1996). Bodies, as reflected in the preoccupations of consumer culture, are at risk from body odour, decaying teeth and gums, spots and blackheads, and may fall prey to numerous other unpleasant and unsociable fates. Moreover, body fluids are perceived as especially threatening of contamination (Laws, 1990). The spread of HIV/AIDS is a recent and powerful reminder of the danger of the body. Here again, individuals have been encouraged by government campaigns and media attention to reform their sexual behaviour and so to escape contamination by other bodies which may carry this deadly virus. Thus the body is also a public health issue and one which requires strict and disciplined maintenance to contain its capacity for contagion.

Bodies have dangerous potential. This is both physical and symbolic. They absorb meaning (Boughton, 1997) and as a system of representations may symbolise dysfunction and disorder. Exploring the link between body images and personhood, Hockey and James (1993) show that individuals with bodies failing to conform to images of the adult body in mainstream culture are not afforded the privileges reserved for those whose bodies do. More than this, bodies which display signs of disorder become subject to attempts to discipline them. Data from within a residential home, cited in Chapter 3 (Hockey, 1990) reveal the centrality of bodily 'cleanliness' within an environment where bodies were gradually transforming themselves into the dead matter of the corpse. For example, bathtimes were logged in a ledger and the bodies and clothing of older people who visited the home for day care were scrutinised for evidence of 'proper' washing habits. In one case an elderly woman in receipt of day care was deeply offended, feeling that she had been coerced into taking baths and given other people's clothes to wear afterwards. 'I wash down every day at home!' she said. And care assistants, in their turn, repeatedly circulated the details of her mild incontinence and her body odour in staff room gossip (ibid.).

Aspects of the living body can therefore be seen to have dangerous potential. The dead body, however, has fulfilled this potential and although bereaved people continue to be emotionally attached to the body of their loved one, there remains, nevertheless, a cultural perception of the corpse as a source of disease and contamination. Furthermore, it represents an indelible loss of self and individuality.

It is the view of the corpse as disordered that provides insight into its handling and treatment in contemporary Western societies. There are two principal features of the modern understanding of the corpse which provide the keys to its management. First, it is the antithesis of the living body within a society where 'life' and 'death' are understood to stand in a dichotomous relationship to one another. Thus, while the social ideals of well-being, sexual attractiveness and fitness are realised via the living body, the corpse is perceived as a symbol of disorder, dysfunction and danger. It is a site of disease and a source of pollution (Prior, 1989; Howarth, 1996). As such, it has become a source of medical knowledge and is seen as requiring professional or expert handling to contain its threat to public health. Second, in increasingly secular societies, the dead body has become the material reality of death; it is the primary signifier of mortality and a key site at which the lost self of the deceased can be represented.

Exploring the social characteristics of the corpse, this chapter will consider the work of morticians – funeral directors and embalmers – in their attempts to combat the disorder wrought by, and within the corpse and to restore the body. The data are drawn from an ethnographic study of funeral directors undertaken in the East End of London in the late 1980s (Howarth, 1996). Morticians work to produce a visual representation of the living person which corresponds to a remembered image of the embodied self of the deceased. While the experience of the self may arise from life, its interconnectedness with other minds means that upon death the body does not immediately lose its social identity. Instead it continues as a site for meaningful relationships between the living and the dead. This perception is central to the work of the undertaker and embalmer for whom the corpse is, initially at least, an object, and moreover, a polluting object. In preparing it for viewing, they seek to decontaminate it while recreating the deceased's personal identity, and to present the body in a life-like fashion. In the backstage regions of the undertaker's premises (Goffman, 1959), the cadaver is an object which is 'worked on' by professionals. However, their work can be seen as a negotiation with the bereaved which has the aim of producing a meaningful and recognisable social being. Employing the language of identity and personality, and projecting desires, such as clothing choice and hairstyle, onto their subjects, they strive to re-humanise the corpse and to create an image of conscious embodiment. In constructing a visual representation or 'memory picture' for their clients, workers are prolonging meaningful contact with the body of the deceased. In this way they too develop a relationship with their dead subjects.

Dysfunction, disorder, danger and pollution

The cadaver has always been a symbol of mortality (Huizinga, 1954). Writing of the Middle Ages, Huizinga noted that *ars moriendi* focused on the decaying body. For example, there remain many tombs dating from that period with transi, or effigies of decaying bodies, lying prostrate. These semi-decomposed bodies, carved in stone, are depicted with worms and insects of the same material. Their purpose was to remind all of the process taking place below. In Christendom these images provided people with a constant reminder that they should not become too attached to this life as all their worldly possessions, including their own bodies, would eventually corrupt and decay. Thus the corpse was simply a reminder of human finitude. Solace came from the priest who preached a Christian belief system which celebrated Christ's triumph over death and allowed good people to look beyond death and to anticipate the life hereafter.

Although in that system the body is a decaying and immoral body, the polluting remains of earthly sin, it nevertheless represents a form of order. It is the natural order of God's universe that all things should die, decay and return to the earth from whence they came – ashes to ashes, dust to dust. In contemporary Western societies the declining role of institutionalised Christianity and the escalation of materialism and individuality have led us to a society where the living body has come to be identified as the site of the self (Synott, 1992). Where once the body was understood to be the vehicle for the soul, it is now afforded central significance in the construction of the self. The loss of mainstream Christian faith has been matched by the force of individualism. In the current system, the dead body is the signifier of the loss of self and the loss of individuality – the material reality of death. As such, the dead body now has a destabilising impact. As Kristeva (1982) argues, the corpse is the abject body, a threat to identity, system and order (see Chapter 2). It is no longer a secure, bounded body. Its orifices threaten to contaminate the external world with internal body matter and fluids; its surfaces cannot be relied upon to remain intact. It has lost its integrity and its wholeness.

Since the nineteenth century, there has developed a physical and symbolic separation between the living and the dead. It was during the last century that the link between disease and hygiene was first established and this, together with the physical separation of the living from the dying and the dead, have led to an increased perception of the corpse as polluting. As illustrated in the previous chapters, pathology assumes that the relationship between death and disease is rooted in the body. 'Death and disease were to be located in the human body, diseases caused death, and the causal sequence which linked the one to the other were made visible in human organs and tissues' (Prior, 1989: 9). If the cause of death is located within the body, then the corpse is not simply a by-product of death but is at once a source of disease and a symbol of mortality. In modern societies, therefore, the dead body is seen as highly polluting: both physically and symbolically. Physical pollution stems from the fear of contamination by disease and decay; symbolic pollution from the fear of mortality and bodily decay, of which the corpse is a signifier.

This view of the dead body as polluting is common to many societies. For example, in Cantonese society, survivors can be contaminated simply by proximity to the corpse or merely by inhaling the 'killing airs' (Watson, 1982). Among the Traveller Gypsies, the immobility of the corpse renders it a highly anomalous – and polluting – entity within a nomadic culture which defines itself in opposition to a mainstream sedentary society. Life finds continuity not in any kind of post-mortem survival or indeed post-mortem memorialisation; rather, life is reproduced in successive generations of Traveller children. The dead, therefore, have no place within Traveller classificatory schema. At the time of death, their ghosts can be dangerous and their bodies are unclean. Traditionally, the trailer in which they lived and died would be burned and their family would move on from the place of illness and death. Since pollution, by definition, adheres to the dominant 'gorgio' culture, deaths now take place in the already 'dirty' space of the gorgio hospital and the dangerous corpse is safely pinned down in the gorgio churchyard (Okely, 1983).

The modern concern with public health, first evident in the nineteenth century, means that the dead have come to be separated from the living and the body of the deceased is removed to the mortuary or chapel of rest. Perceiving the corpse as a source of pollution and a danger to public health has led to a social require- ment for the services of an expert, a professional skilled in negating the corpse's power to contaminate. Morticians utilise pseudo- scientific techniques, such as embalming, to render the corpse harmless to the living. In the *Manual of Funeral Directing*, for example, we find references to science within the terminology used to describe this procedure: 'embalming consists of the injection of a scientifically prepared combination of chemicals into the vascular system of the deceased' (1988: 60). Indeed, the handling of the dead body is usually subject to public health regulations and these rules guide death-workers in decisions pertaining to the appropriate location and sanitisation of the corpse. As a signifier of pollution and a symbol of death, bereaved families in contemporary Western societies normally concede custody to the funeral director who in turn, is, 'prepared to carry out the duty which is the fundamental core of his responsibility, namely, to take into his care and charge the body of the deceased' (NAFD, 1988: 102).

Introducing the concept of embalming to bereaved families, funeral directors adopt the language of preservation and hygiene. The practice is said to afford both psychological and physical protection to their clients as it temporarily preserves human tissue. A primary rationalisation for its use issues from the public health discourse with its concern for the dangers which the decaying body potentially holds for the public. Indeed, the funeral industry in Britain claims of modern arterial embalming that, '[s]ince the treatment destroys all pathogenic bacteria, there is little danger of infection or contagion from an embalmed body' (NAFD, 1988: 59).

It is the embalmer's role to re-establish the body's boundaries. In arresting decomposition and shoring up its physical boundaries, the worker restores the body's social and conceptual boundaries. On the practical level this entails removing the most obvious signs of death which linger, and can be observed on the body. After death the body loses the human qualities associated with vitality: it lacks vigour, the skin becomes discoloured and slack, the hair limp, limbs are stiff and inactive and further deterioration is inevitable as decomposition rapidly erodes the organs and tissues. If the deceased is to regain any semblance of individuality, the decay must be halted, the body preserved, albeit temporarily, and its human features redeemed.

The cadaver is first 'laid out' and this can be carried out by either the undertaker or hospital nurse. The body is washed and finger and toe nails are clipped and cleaned. Men are shaved. The rectum and vagina are plugged with wool. Nostrils are packed if there is discharge, care being taken to avoid altering the contours of the face. Plugs must not be visible. Wounds are sealed (Howarth, 1996).

The mortician may then embalm the body: 'the most powerful weapon in the battle against the corruption of the body' (NAFD, 1988: 59) and undertake the rehabilitation of self-identity. The practice entails draining body fluids from the cadaver and replacing these with formalin – a preservative chemical. A metal rod with a length of tubing attached to it is inserted into the lower abdomen. The rod is then twisted and turned until the body fluids begin to flow out of the body via the tube. The next step is to replenish the emptying vessels with formalin. A small incision is made in the carotid artery at the base of the neck. From here the chemical is pumped into the body. Gentle slapping and massaging of the fingers and lower extremities of the limbs assists the movement of chemical around the body. The chemical revitalises some of the fundamentally human characteristics of the body, transforming the colour of the skin and artificially restoring its elasticity. It also temporarily checks decomposition and so guards against the potential embarrassment of leaking or weeping body surfaces.

By re-establishing the body's boundaries, workers come into direct contact with the most dangerous of the body's polluting products: blood, mucous and excreta. In bolstering up the boundaries of the flesh and presenting the deceased as undamaged and intact, the techniques adopted are themselves violent and transgressing of those very boundaries. The restoration of order therefore needs to be understood as something which operates most powerfully at the symbolic level. In a material sense, the 're-ordered' corpse is one which has undergone mutilation via the invasion of syringes and needles. Lips, for example, will be punctured with needles in order to stitch them into an expression of peace. If the cause of death could be established only after a post-mortem examination, the body will have been systematically fractured – as described in the Chapter 5. Again, the ordering or attribution of meaning to the death – through identification of its cause – occurs, paradoxically, via the radical disruption of the body's integrity. Although not appraised of the details of embalming, some bereaved families may refuse the treatment on the grounds, for example, that, having already undergone considerable surgery, 'she's been cut about enough'. Although in such cases they will respect their clients' wishes, for the mortician, the construction of a body which appears intact, a visual representation of the embodied self, justifies the violence done to it.

Taking custody, the mortician is aware that for the families the body of the deceased is not merely a shell but is vested with memories. As such, it is not an object but a person to whom they retain an emotional attachment. In addition, it is frequently a loved body, a deeply familiar source of comfort which is linked intimately with other bodies: the body of a sexual partner, the body it gave birth to, or the body that gave birth to it. To avoid distressing their clients (and losing business) death-workers must treat their charge with dignity and care. In public at least, they must acknowledge that the body is valuable and entitled to respect. Like the suddenly dead body which the coroner deals with, the disposable body, under the funeral director's jurisdiction, is an ambiguous one. At once profane and sacred, it is an object for the professional; yet for the bereaved, the container of the self. Death-workers perceive themselves as having an obligation to protect their clients from physical pollution and distressing sights, while enabling them to enjoy artificially prolonged meaningful contact with the body of the deceased. Funeral directors deal at a physical, grounded level with death and its boundaries. On a social or conceptual level their work challenges the boundaries between life and death. By transforming the corpse from a defiling object, they simultaneously create a visual representation of its former self; reordering its features and characteristics and presenting it as whole, undamaged and lifelike. As their handbook suggests of embalming:

> [t]his is perhaps the most valuable aspect of the treatment. The change effected is truly remarkable – gone is the deathly pallor and the discoloration of the lower features. Instead the family sees a life-like presentation of their loved one appearing as though peacefully sleeping. The result is a source of great comfort and has a decided psychological value.
>
> (NAFD, 1988: 59)

Visual representations of the embodied self

It was noted earlier that Western cultural images of living bodies are predominantly those of vitality, health and beauty. These representations encompass the notion of individuality – the primary motivating force in their construction. By contrast, the corpse, prior to post-mortem treatment, represents the very opposite of these images – for the body, sacred in life, is profane in death. The dead body lacks health, vitality and beauty, its erstwhile owner having once and for all lost control over its presentation and individuality. Thus the corpse as a symbol of mortality signifies an absence of individuality, a lack of autonomy and irreversible decay. It forces recognition that the personal quest for control and body beautiful is lost. Indeed, it is the perception of the dead body as the antithesis of our aspirations for the living body that amplifies the conviction that the corpse is such a disordered and dangerous object.

Shilling's concept of the 'unfinished body' (1993) encompasses the particular, ongoing project that confronts the individual in modern society: the work of finishing the body through the way in which it is dressed, through the routines of 'hygiene', through exercise and dietary regimes. But the living, material body is always in process. As bodies age, the task of attempting to finish the body becomes more difficult as physical deterioration increasingly betrays or undermines attempts to construct the perfect body. The reconstruction of the body in death is a particularly stark process of finishing, as the body becomes an object to be rescued and returned to an imagined subjectivity. This finishing, however, is not achieved by the individual, as a completed project of self-construction. Rather, it is produced by a stranger, the mortician. In its production, it is frozen in time and, because the self is silent, its meaning and nature can be read only from the surfaces of the body.

In finishing the body, the construction of funeral rites, both preparatory and celebratory, allow the dead body to be transformed into a visual representation of the living one. Mortuary rituals employ a collection of goods and services to convert the corpse, the material reality of death, from an unmanageable spectre into a revitalised or human subject. In so doing, the body becomes a commodity, reconstructed according to the culturally acceptable characteristics of the living body. To achieve this effect, relatives purchase goods such as burial clothes; and services such as embalming and cosmetology, which humanise the cadaver. These act as antidotes to bodily decay, to the threatening image of mortality and to the loss of individuality and self.

Csordas (1994) argues that in everyday life, the body in good health disappears. There is something of a contradiction here, between the taken-for-granted body and the 'unfinished' body as conceptualised by Shilling. However, the bodily project with which we are consumed in life is a project within a defined framework, the limits of which are relatively fixed. Arguably the 'disappearance' of body is one its aims. For example, as Davis notes, women undergoing plastic surgery are not seeking to distinguish themselves as great beauties. Rather they are in pursuit of the invisibility which is granted through possession of an 'ordinary' or 'normal' body (1995, 1997). We can assume, therefore, that in terms of their satisfaction with the work of the surgeon, there is a clearly understood set of criteria which reflect their knowledge of the desirable limits of 'normality'. It is these limits that enable the body to acquire a taken-for-granted nature. With sickness or other major physical transformation, the body once again becomes visible and is objectified by the self – often in terms of an unmanageable or unfamiliar body whose dimensions and possibilities or frailties need to be re-learnt. Turner uses the example of amputation (Turner, 1992). Drawing on Merleau-Ponty's (1962) concept of the lived body and his research with amputees, Turner claims that 'perception and movement can be artificially separated, because basic forms of perception (such as seeing itself) involve body movements' (1992: 43). It is impossible to understand perception without acknowledging that it derives from a particular spatial positioning. For amputees, the loss of a limb shatters the person's spatial awareness and with that comes loss of judgement and perception. The loss of perception is not simply in terms of bodily positioning or movement, but seems likely also to disrupt self-perception or personal identity in that the body not only takes on alien qualities but becomes objectified in the process.

These theoretical perspectives help us to understand the body's visibility in death since it is all that remains of the individual, the self is, temporarily at least, felt to be lost. The loss of the self is accompanied by, or indeed, is evoked by the transformation of the body. The corpse is a silent body and one devoid of other senses. It is cold and unwelcoming. Moreover, as noted earlier in this chapter, it is a potentially dangerous body in that it represents mortality and is in the process of decomposition – a confronting reminder of the fragile and ultimately mortal nature of embodied existence. It is here, with the corpse, that the (re)construction begins; the aim of which is to represent it in a manner which transcends its materiality and re-attaches evidence or signs of self and individuality. It is the mortician, the funeral director or embalmer, who first undertakes the task of identity construction, which may subsequently be developed through the informal talk and practices of surviving friends and family (Walter, 1996). Aspiring to make dead flesh consistent with the living body, morticians employ a variety of technical and cultural devices.

Following embalming, the corpse is subjected to the techniques of restoration and cosmetology. Cotton wool may be packed beneath the eyelids to avoid a sunken appearance. Lips are commonly sewn together to prevent a sagging jaw and are then gently manipulated and smoothed to provide a more natural appearance. If the deceased suffered a violent death and there is substantial damage to the body, the mortician is likely to offer reconstruction work on the body. In cases where there is considerable disfigurement this may require lengthy and intricate work: repairing lacerations, rebuilding facial structures and carefully hiding the scars with make-up. It is only the visible parts of the body which will benefit from this treatment. Although wounds to other parts are sealed prior to embalming, no further restoration will take place as a damaged torso or limbs are easily concealed beneath clothing. The extent to which cosmetics are applied is largely determined by gender. Presuming the cultural norm that women are more likely to wear facial make-up than men, the mortician may use a range of colours and techniques for the former, only adding a little colour to faces of the latter. If considerable restoration was deemed necessary, to the extent where the accuracy of the reconstruction may be at risk, workers may ask the family for a photograph of the dead person.

The final element in reconstructing identity is the presentation and positioning of the body. In displaying the deceased for the benefit of relatives and friends, funeral workers endeavour to produce the impression of a body whose features and constitution closely resemble the living body. When the living body is immobile, if it is not standing or seated it is likely to be at rest, most often asleep. There are cultures which, for the purposes of post-mortem presentation, manipulate the corpse into a seated position (Slobodin, 1997); in contemporary Western societies, it is most likely to be recumbent and resembling a sleeper. The pose should be made to appear natural:

> the head resting on pillows of just the right height, possibly inclined a little to one side...[t]he posing of the arms and hands is also worthy of careful attention for hands can be expressive...A coverlet is supplied so that the finished result is...that of the deceased lying on a divan or bed. The judicious

use of wadding to pack the arms in position can help retain a natural restful posture.

(NAFD, 1988: 57, 63)

Families may provide the funeral director with a set of favourite clothes for the deceased. More frequently, and in keeping with the theme of sleep, the body will be dressed in nightwear. Whatever the design of the clothing, it will be used to hide the secrets of reconstruction, for example, the props which hold the body in particular poses and the scars which undermine the representation of wholeness. Only the head and the hands will be visible, for it is only these parts of the body that are readily accessible in life, and furthermore, it is to these that we look for expression and identity. After treatment by the morticians, visitors who come to view the body are able to comment on the deceased's well-being (Pine, 1975).

The reconstruction, however, is precarious, and having only come to know the body in death, funeral workers may misrepresent the deceased and destroy the illusion of an embodied self. Discontinuity is threatened if the representation is wrong. This is exemplified in the following case.

Following a road accident, an elderly woman was admitted to hospital in a serious condition. Prior to her death, and as part of the attempt to save her life, she received stitching to a deep wound which ran from her hairline to her nose. Her relatives told the funeral director that they were distressed by the sight of the scar this had left on her face when they had seen her in hospital after she had died. The funeral director resolved to reconstruct the woman's face. He removed the stitches, glued the skin together, filled in the blemishes and blended in the skin colour with cosmetics, reconstructing her facial lines and pores. The family's responses to his work were, however, mixed, the restored body yielding a diversity of readings. Thus, while the woman's daughter was thrilled with the work, her granddaughter found the image disturbing, and was unable to reconcile the restored version of the woman's face with the one she had confronted in the hospital. For her, removing the marks of death had disrupted the continuity of the self and thereby undermined her recognition of the representation as her grandmother.

(Howarth, 1996)

The risk involved in attempting to finish the bodily project is that the re-constructed body may project strange or unfamiliar messages. The tint of the skin may not quite match the one produced from the original palette, the hair may be set in a new style, the hands never held like that in life, pyjamas an anathema.

As Lesy (1987, quoted in Ruby, 1995: 12) contends, real death is carefully hidden in our society and transformed into fictionalised images (see Chapter 2). Yet these images or representations are desired by those who consume them. In the death-worker's preparation of the corpse, there is a critically important collusion between the mortician and the family. As Bakhtin argues, social identities are dialogically negotiated (1981), and this is no less the case when it comes to the construction of social identity at the site of the corpse. Workers utilise theatrical techniques to stage the desired image, and families, not searching for the secrets, refuse to look for the props. To raise the coverlet, for example, or to glimpse beneath the body's clothing would destroy the image. Furthermore, in accepting the representation of the body as a subject body, mourners resist the act of peeking since this would violate the boundaries of personal space. They are searching for presence and continuity of identity. This is not to say that they are expecting to see the body as it was in life; but, rather, to view a representation of the dead transformed. They come to witness the body of the loved one rescued from the depths of the profane and inserted into the realm of the sacred, from lost to regained self.

Not all bodies are reconstructed, however. Different bodies hold different meaning. In contrast with the dominant views in contemporary Western societies, there are cultures and religions which perceive of embalming as unnecessary or potentially hazardous to the soul of the deceased. For example, Jehovah's Witnesses resist any intrusive bodily intervention. In cultures such as the Siriono and Hadza the corpse is seen as an irrelevant by-product of death, a shell to be discarded and disposed of with little or no ritual. 'This means that in those societies, discontinuity and individuality is no threat' (Bloch, 1982: 230).

In Chapter 5 we discussed the question of what amounts to a dead body for the purposes of the coroner's inquiry. The 2000-year-old body did not constitute a body whose death required investigation as it lacked any social connection or context and could, therefore, only be recognised and examined as an anatomical object. Given that personal/social identity is constructed in life through social interaction, that is, by reference to others, it is only logical that this should continue to be the case in death. When funeral directors receive a body into their custody, the nature and extent of any reconstruction work will depend on its social connections and cultural meaning. Unless they enjoyed a particularly close relationship, the relatives of an aged aunt, living in a geographically distant town, are unlikely to request that her dead body be prepared for viewing. It is usually only when people expect to continue relationships with the dead, in whatever form, that the body of the deceased is reconstructed to visually recover continuity. For example, in the ostensibly secular society of the USSR, the body of Lenin was embalmed and on permanent public display as a symbol of the continuity of communist ideals.

The British public, indeed the world's public, were not allowed to view the dead body of Diana, Princess of Wales. Her living body had been at the heart of everything that was 'Diana'. Indeed, the complexity of her persona was made most visible in her multiple embodiments: her youthful innocent body, the pregnant body of an expectant mother, the confused and distressed anorexic body, the hairstyle, the clothes, the gym, the cellulite, her sexual relationships, her unclothed body. Through the cameras of the media, Diana's body became a publicly familiar body, the changing contours of which reflected developments in her social and personal life and were topics for public and private debate. The scrutiny of her body ceased with her death, as it disappeared behind icons of regal and national identity – the gun carriage, the uniformed military personnel and the Union Jack. It was only through illicit photographs, reflecting a fascination with the vulnerable body, that a handful of images of her dying and dead body surfaced. The circulation of these photographs was popularly viewed with disgust and contempt, the content and detail of her injuries and medical treatment listened to with horror. Her body, so familiar, glamorous and desirable in life, disappeared from public view in death. She was the epitome of vitality and, therefore, perhaps she could not be represented in death. She was larger than life. The same was said of Marilyn Monroe at the time of her death, and, as Elton John sang, '[a]ll the papers had to say was that Marilyn was found in the nude'.

At a more mundane level, the bodies of those who die without relatives or close friends also disappear from view. They will be unceremoniously coffined and cremated with only a minimally religious service. The public purse does not stretch to reconstruction and, moreover, given the lack of social contacts there is no obvious need. It is not only in the secular Western society of today that the bodies of the destitute are culturally perceived as having less value. The Anatomy Act of 1832, enacted at a time when the condition of the physical body was still popularly believed to contribute to its progress in the afterlife, made provision for the bodies of the poor who died in workhouses to be surrendered to the surgeons and anatomists as objects for dissection (Richardson, 1987). If in death the poor escaped the surgeon's knife, their bodies would normally have been buried in a pauper's grave. These graves, and the mass graves of the victims of genocide in which the dead have lost their individuality, tend to be viewed with the utmost horror and dread. Worse than the fate of the mass grave is the absence of any grave at all because bodies have been lost. Indeed, much of the horror relayed by the men who survived World War I stems from the loss and dismemberment of bodies. Beyond that, many appear to have been severely traumatised by their own ability, indeed by the necessity, to dehumanise the bodies and fragments of bodies, which formed a constituent part of trench warfare. After the war in an effort to restore dignity the War Graves Commission employed 15,000 men to exhume and re-inter the bodies of the dead. In the desire to recover as many bodies as possible, 'the whole battlefield area in France and Flanders was searched six times, some parts as many as 29 times' (Hammerton, undated: 7892).

The disposal of the body

Once the body has been ritually viewed and the required amount of time has lapsed since the death, it will be disposed of, either by cremation or burial. The reconstruction and the arrest of decomposition which makes the body safe, are temporary phenomena. Like all theatrical performances, they are not designed to last; they are not real but illusion and when the time comes for the performance to close, the body must be disposed of. The ritual reconstruction of the body as a container of the self has provided the memory picture and for the bereaved family and friends this has facilitated a prolongation of their meaningful contact with the deceased. Although these post-mortem procedures have only temporary impact, the illusory effect is sufficient because the practice of humanisation is not a denial of death but an extension of the self. To allow the material body to remain any longer would be to invite instability, to risk a failed performance and to encourage disorder. The body would, in Douglas' terms, constitute matter out of place (Douglas, 1966). The ordering of the body, and the appropriate sequencing of treatment for the corpse, therefore culminates in its disposal. In this way, the illusion of a post-mortem continuity of self-identity is sustained. This contrasts with the practices of Traveller Gypsies, discussed above, where the dangerous dead must be dispersed (Okely, 1983). Rather than committing to memory the beautified face of a loved one, Traveller Gypsies will press their open hands across its features with the aim of *forgetting* the image. Lesser contact carries the risk that the memory of the face will haunt the living.

For many members of Western society, including Traveller Gypsies themselves, once the corpse has been properly disposed of, it no longer represents a danger. In mainstream society, the site of disposal may become a place of pilgrimage for the bereaved, but the material body is without any further social role. There is a clear distinction between being dead and being buried. Once buried, the focus for survivors turns to their memories of the deceased and the ongoing presence of the person in their lives. For many cultures the dead ancestors play their part in watching over, protecting and bringing good fortune to the lives of those left behind (Bloch, 1971; Watson, 1982).

In Western societies cremation, at around 67 per cent of all disposals, has become more popular than burial (Jupp, 1990). A number of reasons have been suggested for this: more efficient use of space, the impact of greater geographical mobility and therefore the breakdown of traditional family responsibility for caring for the grave, and a popular belief that cremation is 'cleaner' and avoids the risk of future contamination from human remains decomposing in the earth. If buried, however, the bodies of the dead should remain undisturbed in their resting place. They should, as gravestones frequently remind us, 'Rest In Peace'. The disturbance of human remains is generally viewed with horror as the unlawful 'resurrection' of the abhorrent dead. Literature and film fantasies of Egyptian mummies and partially decomposed zombies returning from the dead at once fascinate and repel the audience. The reality of exhumation holds similar tensions as the act of disinterring a body carries a range of social and cultural significances. Bodies can be exhumed for legal reasons: the coroner has the power to disinter remains for the purpose of holding an inquest. A religious meaning can be attached to the act of exhumation if a body is being moved from one burial to another, from unconsecrated to consecrated ground. It can hold nationalistic meaning as in the disinterment of the corpse of the 'unknown soldier' and its relocation in a cenotaph. It can carry meanings of community identity and political struggle for the recognition of ethnic groups as in the case of the relocation of the bodies of Aboriginal people buried in distant or alien burial grounds – a homecoming. A related example is the University of Nebraska's agreement to return the remains which it held of 1,700 American Indians, material which had been used for the study of early Americans. Since the precise tribal affiliation of the remains could not be determined, they were all to be interred on the land of the nearby Omaha tribe. Allen Hare of the Sioux tribe is reported as saying that 'The unaffiliated remains all come from Mother Earth. They should be returned to nourish the soil, bring food to people' (*The Higher*, 25 September 1998). The exhumation of bodies can also be a political weapon as in the case of the Republican exhumation of the bodies of priests and nuns during the Spanish Civil War (Lincoln, 1993) (see Chapter 2). The powerful Church was viewed by the Republicans as having imposed its tyrannical rule over the poor for centuries. The exhumation of the bodies of its saints was therefore a deliberate act of defilement, the public exhibition of their decomposing remains being designed to expose the corrupt nature of the Church.

Conclusion

We have argued that the construction of meaning at the site of body can intensify in specific ways after a death. This chapter has shown how the body in death can be made to reflect the social preoccupation with the body in life. Indeed, it is argued here, that in modern Western societies, preoccupied as we are with the living body and its properties of vitality, there continues to be tremendous difficulty and fear entailed in confronting the dead body as a material entity which abrogates the powerful cultural drive for the body beautiful, healthy and youthful.

The corpse is perceived as physically polluting and one aim of the mortician is to shield clients from contamination. As the material reality of death, the body is also symbolically threatening as it represents discontinuity, disorder and mortality. At an individual level it signals loss of identity. When living bodies fail, there are attempts, either by the individual, professionals or carers, to revitalise their physical functioning and to restore order and stability to dishevelled or disorderly flesh. Similar attempts are made by funeral and embalming professionals who strive to reconstruct the corpse in ways that project bodily order, continuity of meaning and prolongation of identity: a visual representation of its former self. The illusion depends for its success on client collusion. Bereaved people, like the audience at a theatre, attend the viewing in order to suspend reality. While they pay their respects to a mother, husband or son, they are not unaware that what they can see and touch is a corpse. We argue, therefore, that surviving family and friends come to witness the reconstruction or silent resurrection of the deceased person. Indeed, as their comments reveal, there is a sense in which they come to admire the funeral director and the embalmer's scientific 'craft'. 'Doesn't he look well' is a response which should not be taken as evidence that family are failing to recognise that the 'person' laid out before them has suffered serious illness or injury. Rather, we suggest, they are expressing appreciation of the restorative arts of the professional.

As we have indicated, not all bodies are reconstructed. Without the appropriate social context, the representation of the deceased at the site of the body carries no meaning. Some bodies have lost social connection and without an 'audience', the 'performance' of identity cannot be played out; other bodies have strong social links but are themselves lost, buried anonymously in mass graves, and some bodies are never buried. These unreconstructed and radically unfinished bodies haunt the imaginations of survivors. Rather than maintaining intimate social relationships with the dead, family and friends may be dogged by a fear that the dead and decomposing body will return, uninvited.

Chapter 8

Married life after death

Embodiment and self

If we submit to a growing intellectual demand that we take account of the embodied nature of human life in our attempts to make sense of the social world, it is the dead body which most powerfully confronts us with the question of what social scientists understand by the term 'human life'. When posed, this question often materialises as 'what is it that constitutes the self?'. We need to recognise this question as one which has emerged from a quite specific Western intellectual heritage. Asad argues that it was during the seventeenth century that self-reference began to beckon as Descartes equated the human mind with consciousness (1998). The religious imperative to care for, or save, oneself lies at the roots of the notion of the 'subject' and by the late eighteenth century the mind had come to be understood as the subject within which ideas inhere. The possibility of the self or ego had come into being. It is therefore a socio-historically specific concept – 'self' – which underpins a recent focus on the embodied nature of selfhood within social theories of the body. And indeed this concept – 'self' – has close allies in a set of kindred terms; identity, personhood, and the individual, all of which are quite specific to our own socio-cultural moment. Within this model of the self, flesh becomes central to a process described by Bryan Turner as 'enselvement' (1998). When the flesh ceases to be, when it is cremated or when it rots, we are left with the question of how 'self' and 'flesh', as conceived of by social scientists, actually relate to one another. If self and body are identical or mutually constitutive, does this mean that the self is discontinuous, something which is repeatedly reinvented as change takes place within and on the body's fleshly surfaces? If this is the case, is the self entirely dissipated once the body has been pronounced dead?

While this may seem like a question which only religious thinkers are qualified to ask – 'Is there a life after death?' – in this, and the following two chapters of the book, we show why social scientists also need to explore it. To date, however, they have tended to limit their task to the identification and representation of the beliefs of others as to how self and body relate to one another. Here we suggest that we need to go further in our theoretical thinking in order to be clear about who or what is encompassed within our models of the social world. Without an explicit account, we risk developing a theoretical orientation towards this question which merely replicates the belief system of our particular socio-historical moment.

Producing selves

In previous chapters we have examined sets of practices which allowed the self to be made to inhere within the dead body, recognising that selfhood is precarious, even for those who are embodied, for example, for the 'vegetables' who lie among drips and catheters in hospital side wards; and for the unbounded hospice bodies whose 'self appears to have "gone" altogether, leaving little, if anything, but the "empty" body' (Lawton, 1998: 130). Through the work of funeral directors and embalmers, however, the self can be reconstituted at the site of the dead body. Flesh, even when dead, therefore remains a key prop within the production of 'self', albeit in a fashion which on some level we find disturbing – and we may find ourselves concurring with Evelyn Waugh (1948) and Jessica Mitford's (1963) debunking of the funeral director's products. In the chapters which follow, however, we question the view that the disposal of the body brings social being to an end. Older widows and widowers, for example, may continue to enjoy significant social relationships with their 'dead' spouse. Rather than a materiality which is limited to the body itself, material objects and phenomena such as clothing and significant sounds, sights and smells associated with the former partner begin to take on new resonances for bereaved people. Indeed, contact with the dead is not unusual among bereaved people. For some this is a spontaneous experience; for others is achieved through the services of informal ritual specialists such as clairvoyants. As will be argued, their practices can be seen as an attempt to incorporate the dead within the social world – one which involves bringing them to hand. This contrasts with the practices of Christian clergy which also represent a belief in 'life' beyond embodiment, but one which creates clear sets of distances between the living and the dead and indeed discourages individualised communication between them.

Agency, self and embodiment

Predominant within current social theories of the body is a focus on human agency, expressed most typically in the post-traditional project of self-construction. In the conditions of high modernity, therefore, we catch the embodied self at work, free to constitute itself along the lines of its own choice, but adrift among the competing authorities of fashion, science, medicine and the media. None the less, this agency, expressed in tasks of bodily self-construction such as health care, fitness regimes and plastic surgery, can be seen merely as the individual resisting the body's constraints and limitations in a spurious attempt to deflect awareness from its inevitably mortal nature (Bauman, 1992). This theoretical orientation towards the embodied self – or enselvement – is not one which readily incorporates the ageing, dying and dead body. It rests upon a conception of agency as body-based, with human flesh as the site and source of individualised, intentional action within the world. The body in crisis therefore challenges this easy elision of agency, enselvement and flesh and demands a re-appraisal of the assumptions which currently underpin social theories of embodiment.

Asad (1998) argues that our prevailing conceptions of agency stem from a particular theoretical project or agenda. That is, they reflect a concern to limit the potency of the concept of structure. By differentiating between social structure and individual experience, early social scientists were able to identify for themselves a field of study – 'society'. In Durkheimian terms, it was something which existed over and above the sum of its individual members and so provided a legitimate disciplinary focus. However, this reified notion of macro-level structures of power offers few theoretical resources for the study of micro-level experience or indeed the processes of social change. It is therefore with the aim of redressing this imbalance that a very particular conception of agency has come into being, namely, the intentional power of society's individual members to act not just within but also upon the structures of their social world.

Agency, in this sense, is something which social scientists attribute to the human behaviour which they study, a way of making human accidents into necessities which misleadingly combines cause with effect (Asad, 1998). It is too sure-footed, Asad suggests, as a way of framing human action. Indeed, it evokes the way health promotion policies assume individuals to be agents who will act rationally on their own behalf; that is, people who consciously and deliberately pursue health maintaining practices at the cost of other agendas and priorities (Nettleton, 1998).

However, it is not just a model of agency which attributes a spuriously rational intentionality to society's individual members; it is also a model of agency which is limited to the actions of human beings. In its place, Assad substitutes a formulation of agency as things or persons who make a difference, of empowerment at particular sites. His suggestion is echoed by Prout who draws on Latour's work to argue that, 'agency is an effect brought about by the assembly of heterogeneous materials. It is produced through the connections between an empirically diverse set of resources; discursive, biological, technological and so on' (forthcoming).

In contrast to the arguments put forward by these authors, therefore, the more limited notion of agency which underpins many social theories of embodiment emerges as a formulation of ideas which is highly specific to dominant Western agendas. This is brought out via cross-cultural comparison, as in Becker's work on body, self and society in Fiji (1995). Her observations of the cultivation of social relationships, largely expressed through nurturing and food exchange, revealed a vested interest in cultivating others' bodies rather than one's own. On the basis of this material she formulated a notion of agency as a collective phenomenon: 'bodily experience transcends the individual body, is diffused to other bodies, and is even manifest in the environment' (ibid.: 127). She goes on to say that 'the self...whilst certainly connected to its body, is not its exclusive agent' (ibid.). Csordas offers a parallel example from Leenhardt's work among the New Caledonian Peoples where, again, the body was not individuated but 'diffused with other persons and things in a unitary sociomythic domain' (1994: 7). Finally, Battersby highlights the masculinist bias within contemporary Western conceptions of the self and its agency. Her work reminds us that even within a specific socio-historical moment there may well be a diversity of experience, masked by the hegemony of a particular set of models. Responding to Johnson's work on the use of a container as a model or metaphor for the body/self, she says, 'as I read Johnson's and Lakoff's accounts of embodiment, I register a shock of strangeness: of wondering what it would be like to inhabit a body like that' (1993: 31). The model which she feels more at home with is one which reflects a dissipative or inter-subjective self; 'not all talk of identity involves thinking of the self as unitary or contained; nor indeed need boundaries be conceived in ways that make the identity closed, autonomous or impermeable' (ibid.: 38).

Here we argue that many of the social scientists who address society's dead members in their work limit themselves to a model of agency which assumes individual, intentional and embodied action as a prerequisite for social being. From this perspective, the dead are social beings only to the extent that other people – their families, friends or subjects – believe them to be. They exist purely in a psychological sense, within the minds and memories of those who survive them. Just as women previously had a social class position only by virtue of their husbands' jobs, so the dead have social being only by virtue of their survivors' belief systems. Challenging this approach, we argue that a narrow but dominant model of agency currently obscures the dead from the sociological gaze. It mirrors the empiricist, materialist models which lie at the core of Western thought and experience. These relegate the dead to peripheral religious practices and the pathologised longings of lonely widows. Without muscles to flex, tongues to speak or fists to shake, the dead become nothing more than memories which are locked within the imaginations of others.

The remaining chapters of this book set out to develop a theoretical framework which rescues the dead from the obscurity of their survivors' skulls. It examines a range of material which suggests that we need to accord the dead a much fuller social presence than is customary within Western scientific frameworks of knowledge. It is a range of material which also demands a re-evaluation of the notion of agency as it is often understood among social scientists.

In her work on spirit possession, Mary Keller (1998) argues that this is an area which challenges the idea of religion as a belief system housed within the psychology of the individual. Instead, spirit possession requires us to consider religion as a constitutive process or set of embodied practices. Indeed, Keller points out the contradictions of a social theory which, though highlighting the potency of embodied practice, still divides the body from the mind and situates belief within the psyche of the individual – particularly if that belief lies outside the materialist frameworks which predominate within Western societies. For her the efficacy or instrumental agency of a spirit is indivisible from the body of the person possessed. Their body becomes like a flute which is being played. Thus, she does not restrict her understanding of possession to a set of behaviours which represent or symbolise something other, such as a set of beliefs or aspects of a wider social and economic structure. Instead, she argues, what is taking place has an intrinsic social reality or effect as a set of embodied practices taking place within a particular spatio-temporal locality.

It is the direction offered by her work which we intend to follow here, neither engaging with questions as to whether or not the dead are actually 'real' nor relegating them to the margins of a grief-stricken psyche. Instead we focus on three case study areas: widowhood in later life, Christian exorcism, and clairvoyance. They allow us to develop an account of society which incorporates its dead members, using a model of agency not just as a property of the full-bodied individual but, more broadly, as empowerment at a particular site.

The continuing presence of the dead in the lives of elderly widows

This chapter will consider the phenomenon of the continuing presence of the dead in the lives of survivors. It takes as its focus elderly widows and asks, to what extent does married life continue after the biological death of a spouse? In choosing to examine the experience of elderly widows the intention is not to diminish the significance of other relationships that continue after death; those, for example, between parent and child. Rather, this emphasis facilitates the exploration of relationships that elderly, and sometimes socially dead survivors may experience with a biologically dead partner. The data drawn on in this chapter derive largely from in-depth interviews conducted with elderly widows in London in 1993–4. This work was carried out as part of a study funded by the Nuffield Foundation which examined quality of life among older adults living independently in the community.

Widowhood is a gendered experience; differential mortality rates between men and women mean that women, on average, live longer than men (Arber and Ginn, 1991). Given that there is still a cultural norm for women to marry older men, it is therefore, more likely, that if a marriage is to survive biological death, it will more commonly exist between a dead male and a bereaved female spouse.

As noted earlier, there is a body of literature which addresses the concept of social death (see Chapter 3). Social death occurs when a person, whether or not biologically dead, ceases to be treated 'as an active agent in the ongoing social world' of some other person or persons (Mulkay, 1993: 33). According to this definition, social death may occur before, at, or after biological death. Indeed the biological death of a spouse may initiate the social death of the widow. There are cultures in which women become marginal to the life of the community subsequent to the death of their husband (Bowker, 1991). In contemporary Western societies widowhood may be experienced by some women as a form of liberation, after which they are no longer subject to their husband's demands. For others, bereavement may lead to social death as the widow is excluded from 'coupled' social groups and from social networks which rely on the presence of a partner. Indeed, in very old age, and especially for people who are housebound, partners may effectively have become the sole source of social life. Membership of a wider social network can wither away, even before one or other partner has died. In these cases the death of a spouse, particularly for women who are expected to be able to cope alone with the practicalities of independent living, may result in a sudden or severe transition to a state of social death. Their situation can be contrasted with widowers who are more likely to receive an influx of social and practical support, either professional or informal (Howarth, 1995).

While widows may find themselves undergoing some form of social death, they may also continue a relationship with their biologically dead spouse. For social death does not necessarily coincide with biological death. Adopting the definition stated earlier, social death depends upon the extent to which an individual continues to be an active agent in the lives of others. As Mulkay points out, '[s]ocial life is the obverse of social death and depends on the social continuation of the particular person, whether or not that person is biologically alive' (1993: 33). A person whose physical body is dead may therefore continue to have an active presence in the lives of others. While remaining socially present within the life of one person, however, the deceased may be very much dead for another as the nature of social existence depends on interaction. A widow, for example, may pursue social interaction with a spouse where a son, daughter or sibling may not. For the widow, the deceased remains socially alive, has a continued presence and, furthermore, may exert influence on the nature and direction of her life. The extent to which the dead make themselves felt by the living depends in part on the degree to which the living invite them to do so. When the dead are no longer required to participate in social life, when they have ceased to be active agents, then they may become socially dead. However, in other cases, the dead can be seen to retain the powerful but unwelcome influence which they exercised throughout life. Here we focus primarily on the former case.

Continuing presence

Partners may be talked to, or talked about. Self-help groups have been shown to offer a forum where bereaved people are allowed to keep the dead alive; a place where they can share their experiences with similar others and escape the imperative to leave the dead behind and get on with life (Klass, 1984; Riches and Dawson, 1997; Rock, 1997). Anniversaries, birthdays and death-days may be celebrated, marking the passage of time and perhaps adding to the number of years of marriage.

Objects furnish links with the deceased. A dead man's possessions and clothing can bring the partners closer. Elderly widows wearing their husband's sweaters may not simply be keeping warm or saving money but utilising the object to continue the link with the dead spouse. Photographs of the dead, displayed in prominent positions in the home also encourage presence. Photographs on gravestones not only remind those with intimate knowledge, but also inform the stranger, about the body of the deceased as it was in life. They challenge the observer to recognise and endorse the portrait above the tomb rather than to dwell on the decaying matter below.

Sometimes the widow may actually see the dead partner, as he was in life. At other times, and for other people, the husband's presence may be invoked by sounds, sights or smells; a piece of music, the sound of footsteps on the staircase, the sensation of a light breeze unexpectedly caressing her face, a few lines from a letter, the scent of roses. Among widows attending training sessions for bereavement counselling work, there was a shared recognition of the experience of 'feeling the bed go down' with the weight of a partner's body, despite their absence in embodied form.

Unlike spiritualism or clairvoyance, the nature of these widows continuing communication with their dead spouses was usually spontaneous and involved direct rather than mediated interaction. Moreover, it did not take the form of a single, spectacular or dramatic incident or visitation, but rather, it became a mundane series of taken-for-granted interactions, remarkable only to the extent to which they reflected 'normal' social relationships.

The dead may also appear in dreams.

> And sometimes I say to my husband, 'Why can't you help me?'. I used to dream about him a lot....But he used to say to me, 'Stop pulling the covers off me, Doll.' And I used to say, 'I'm not.' I'd answer him back and when I put my arm out he wasn't there. Another thing he'd say is, 'Where's the boys?' And I'm dreaming it. And I'd still answer him. I'd say, 'Well they've gone out together.' When I used to look round I thought where is he?
>
> (Howarth, 1994)

Some of the women interviewed reported hearing their husbands call their name, and others spoke to them in their subconscious. Some would actually talk with their husbands to elicit the answer to a question or to gain a sense of direction. Survivors would look to the dead spouse for advice. This could take the form of anticipating the partner's response to a problem. Whatever the nature of the interaction, the husband continued to play an active part in the woman's life, providing a benchmark against which proposed action can be assessed.

Husbands could also provide companionship. They might appear in the familiar environment of the home, seated in a favourite chair, quietly passing the evening: 'I sit here often and I can see my husband sitting there. I know he's there, he's here' (Howarth, 1994).

These forms of presence are evidence of the continued social existence of the dead in the lives of the living, with dead husbands impacting on the daily lives of survivors. But if the self is constituted via the flesh (Turner, 1998), how can the self survive as an active agent once the physical body has gone? We argue here that if we adhere to the notion that the self has agency and that agency inheres in the self, then biologically dead people who continue as active agents in the lives of the living have retained a form of self. This analysis highlights the inter-subjective nature of the self. The self is constructed through interaction and is inextricably bound up with the selves of others. Although the death of a significant person, whether loved or hated, results in a loss to the self, for a woman whose husband dies, the activities and experiences with which she engaged as his partner may be inseparably intertwined with her own sense of self. There may be no clear boundary between her-self and his-self. This challenges the modern and masculine notion that the bodies of individuals are bounded, exclusive containers of the self; separate from, and unadulterated by the bodies and selves of others. In relationships that extend beyond biological death, the body of the widow is intimately connected with the self of the dead husband. His continued social existence is not psychological, occurring solely within the head of the survivor. Rather, his presence is experienced through physical contacts that re-establish intimate connections. They engender embodied sensations and may stimulate physiological responses: a sense of calm, bodily warmth, comfort, or at the other end of the spectrum, the physical pain that can result from the absence of the other's physical body. These sensations are experienced through the living body and its senses. Although the physical body of the dead partner is absent, his presence is experienced through and within the body of the widow, via feelings and senses such as sight, sound, smell, touch. The senses link individuals to the external world and facilitate contact with it. The experience of the continuing presence of biologically dead partners, therefore, is not located solely in the mind, it is not an illusion or delusion, the widow is not confused and cannot be said to have taken leave of her senses. Accepting Asad's (1998) understanding of agency as empowerment at a particular site, the agency of the biologically dead man is located within the body of the living woman and is indivisible from it. The woman's body is the site of empowerment. The continuing relationship is, in Csordas' terms (1994), one of shared dialogical physicality.

The enduring communion between widow and spouse rejects the temporal and spatial boundaries between the living and the dead. These continued relationships, however, are hedged in with ritual and moral boundaries. As noted above, they are perceived as destabilising the boundaries of the self. They also challenge the binary divisions between life and death and, as such, threaten social stability. On a popular level they may be interpreted as a refusal to 'let go', selfishly extending the life of the deceased and refusing to allow them to 'rest in peace'. On another level, this failure to give up the dead is perceived as psychologically negative, medically pathological.

Medicalised grief

Grief and bereavement have become medicalised. Medical models of bereavement, whether phase (Bowlby, 1980; Parkes, 1986), task (Worden, 1991), or process (Rando, 1992), insist that a healthy outcome can only be achieved once the survivor has emotionally detached themselves from the dead. The dominant discourse which recommends that bereaved people relinquish cross-dimensional relationships is a medical one which relies on the metaphor of healing. The scars of loss will be repaired once the deceased has been properly relocated. This entails 'coming to terms' with the death. On the understanding that it will help them become reconciled to the fact of death, survivors are frequently encouraged to visit the funeral home to view the dead body. This is somewhat paradoxical when we consider the lengths to which funeral directors go to present the corpse as 'lifelike' (see Chapter 7). In accepting that the person is dead, the healing process then moves forward by encouraging the living to re-order their social relationship with the deceased, gradually withdrawing emotional ties. In so doing they are not expected to forget the person, but to allocate them a place in their memory. This memory is retrospective, fixed in time and space. It is not prospective, dynamically anticipating future interaction. To continue communication with the dead is viewed as a pathological desire to live in the past and a barrier to reinvesting emotional energy in new relationships. 'Mourning cannot be complete unless the bereaved succeed in making an adequate worldly adjustment without the one they have lost' (Hinton, 1967: 185). There is an assumption here that meaningful relationships are monogamous and zero-sum; that it is not possible to establish a new relationship without giving up an old one. Moreover, relationships which breach the divide between this world and beyond are perceived as fundamentally disordered and immoral.

Resisting the dominant discourse

Despite the potency and prevalence of medicalised models of grief, as we have argued of other spheres of human embodiment, there is resistance to this dominant model. Indeed, underlying the medical discourse of detachment may be a popular, more traditional discourse which upholds the practice of maintaining associations with the dead. Indeed, it seems probable that the living have always conducted relationships with the dead (Gillis, 1997). For example, the Sora of India continue relationships with the dead through dialogue mediated by the shaman (Vitebsky 1990).

> Almost all societies, it seems, believe that, despite a bodily death, the person not only lives on but continues his relationships with the living, at least for a time. In many cultures these relationships are conceived as wholly beneficial.
>
> (Bowlby, 1980: 123)

Mulkay (1993) suggests that families in Western societies have always retained a bond with the dead and, in Victorian society in particular, it was women who helped to extend their social existence by commemorating birthdays, visiting the grave, and conducting regular prayers. We might add to this that women assumed large responsibility for publicly expressing grief by attiring their bodies in mourning clothing and jewellery. While acknowledging loss, these practices also 'served as mechanisms to extend the social existence of the deceased' (ibid.: 40). In this analysis the distinction between life and death is not so sharp and Mulkay argues that women spent 'much of their lives in the borderland between life and death' (ibid.: 40). Gillis (1997) supports this position, contending that the rise of spiritualism in the mid-nineteenth century reflected a lessening of the distance between the living and the dead: 'the living and the dead existed in the same spatial and temporal continuum' (ibid.: 218). In terms of the family, he argues that the dead are part of the extended, imagined family and he perceives a refusal to allow the dead to depart. They are instead kept alive through linking objects such as photographs, mementos, burial grounds, and more recently, home-made videos and cremated ashes.

One of the key sites within which the social 'life' of the dead takes place is the cemetery and indeed they are often referred to as the cities of the dead. As Kellaher *et al.* (1998) show, like friends and relatives in any other city, the dead can be visited, alone or in company, brought flowers, communicated with, said goodbye to, and revisited. Over time the cemetery has played a significant role in grief and has offered bereaved people a physical place to locate their dead. From the nineteenth century onwards, however, this space became separated, physically and symbolically, from that allocated to the living. More recently, in many European and in Australian societies, cremation has become the preferred method of disposal. In the United Kingdom around 70 per cent of people choose cremation (Jupp, 1993). Cremation has been popularised for a number of reasons. It is assumed to be more sanitary and of less risk to public health; greater geographical mobility has resulted in families having less time to tend and care for graves; it is less expensive and does not take up land that might be used for the living. Indeed, cremation eliminates the need to allocate space for the dead. Although relatives may be invited to bury the ashes of the deceased in a 'rose garden' and to use that place as a focus for memorial, this is rarely successful as their rose is a rose among many other roses, clustered together in an undifferentiated fashion without a headstone identifying the deceased and the survivors who visit the site. Alternatively, families may discard the ashes, leaving them at the disposal of the crematorium, who, after a fixed time and reminder letters, may scatter the ashes in the crematorium grounds. More often, bereaved people will choose to scatter the ashes themselves, in some cases employing the liturgical services of a priest. This scattering might be in the crematorium grounds or at a local beauty spot, a favourite park, water-view, into the seas, or in their own garden, perhaps buried under a plant. Others may keep the ashes in the home, perhaps in a pot on the mantlepiece (Gorer, 1965). The point is that the cremated dead no longer have a fixed place. In one sense they are nowhere. In another sense they may be everywhere. Graves contain the encoffined dead. Cremation allows them mobility and the potential opportunity to continue social relations with the living.

In contemporary society, though, these relationships or connec- tions with the dead have become less visible, concealed by the dominant discourse which disparagingly defines them as either hallucinations, transitory, adaptational phenomena or pathological aberrations. While individuals do continue communion with the dead, they are unlikely to publicise these relationships for fear of being labelled as pathological or complicated grievers, whether by their GPs or more distant family members. In their view, the dead are to be left behind and objects which link the living with the dead, such as clothing and personal possessions should be cleared from the home.

Ontological security and biographical narrative

When a partner dies, especially after a relationship that has spanned many years, the world of the survivor may be thrown into turmoil. In order to regain ontological security the individual must construct a biographical narrative which not only restores a sense of meaning but also provides continuity. In order to move forward to the future, they must have a clear sense of who they are in the present and of how the past has led them to that present. The place of the deceased in the narrative can be highly significant. Research now demonstrates that bereaved people do not normally locate the dead in a past or earlier biography, but that they take the dead with them in the ongoing narrative of their lives (Klass *et al.*, 1996). Marwit and Klass (1994), for example, suggest that bereaved people construct 'inner representations' of the deceased which they carry with them. While this analysis usefully develops the idea that the dead remain socially alive, here we argue that the dead not only live in an 'inner' or psychological sense but, more consequentially, in a social sense, exercise agency within the lives of survivors. Furthermore, we suggest that this continued existence is experienced by survivors in an embodied manner through their own bodies and biological senses.

The continued presence of the dead may be regular and frequent. Indeed, socially isolated elderly women may actually be enjoying better quality relationships with the dead than with the living (Mulkay, 1993). These continued relationships, however, between widow and husband, are not static, fixed in time and based solely on the nature of interaction in life. Rather, they are dynamic relationships within which survivors develop new forms of interactions and, as their life changes, they craft new relationships with the living and with the dead. Immediately following the death of a husband, the bond they share may be particularly strong. Her connection with him is reinforced in her redefined status as widow, that is, as the surviving partner of the dead husband. Moreover, as Moss and Moss (1996) note, if the woman is financially reliant on her husband's pension her tie with him is perpetually reinforced. As Rees (1971) noted, the relationship between the elderly widows and their dead partners can continue for years.

Relationships may, however, become less intense if the widow has or develops more significant relationships with the living. Shortly after the death of a spouse, an elderly woman may seek assistance and support from her husband, complying with the advice given and anticipating the manner in which the husband may have behaved in similar situations. As time goes by and the woman becomes more confident in her own ability to make decisions, she may seek advice less frequently. Furthermore, she may *follow* the advice less frequently, now at liberty to openly disagree with her husband's interpretations. If a widow decides to remarry she may feel more comfortable with this decision if she has 'a sense of permission from the deceased spouse' (Moss and Moss, 1996: 169). While it is not always possible to keep faith with the dead, it is possible to move on and to retain the relationship with the dead, albeit in a new form. The new marriage may then exist within a triadic framework which encompasses the two dyadic relationships the woman enjoys with both her husbands.

Whether or not remarriage occurs, the frequency, location and nature of the communication with the deceased may change. The relationship may develop into one where the woman exerts the greatest amount of control, enjoying it on her own terms. As an interactive relationship it may even disappear altogether.

Reconstitution and discontinuities

It is not simply the case, however, that the living are retaining bonds with the dead. As noted earlier, the dead may also seek to continue their social presence, some, even imposing themselves where they are not wanted.

In having greater awareness of their status as dying (Field, 1996), people are able to prepare their legacy for those they leave behind. In wills people leave possessions which they hope will continue to locate them in the social lives of survivors. Matthews (1979) showed

that elderly women bequeathed personal and meaningful belong-
ings such as jewellery in order to cheat death and retain a social
presence. Writing letters to be opened after death and the
production of personal videos containing messages for the living,
can also be interpreted as attempts by the dying to reconstitute
themselves after death. Mechanisms such as these encourage
ongoing communication, the dead projecting themselves into a
future that they will not experience.

But not all survivors desire to continue relationships with the
dead. For elderly widows, the relationship in life may not have been
harmonious or pleasurable. Some women quickly forget their
partners; others would leave them behind if only they were able.
Bennett (1985) notes the existence of the 'good dead', those who
confirm and comfort the living. It is worth noting that the dead
spouse may not necessarily have a comforting presence. Post-
mortem relationships may be stormy, as they were in life, perhaps
involving both pleasure and pain. The continued presence of the
husband may not be confirming; may never have been so. In some
cases the widow may be relieved that her husband is dead.

> He was an alcoholic and when he came home he'd hit me. I
> stayed with him for the sake of the children and because we had
> nowhere else to go. By the time they'd grown up and left home
> it was too late to think of starting again. And as he got older
> and ill, he calmed down a bit. But I never forgot or forgave. I
> suppose I shouldn't say this but I was glad when he died.
>
> (Howarth, 1994)

This woman did not continue the relationship with her husband
after death. Indeed, his continued presence would have been
distressing to her. It would seem, then, that in modern societies
continued relationships are more a matter of the personal choice of
the living. Unlike the relationships with ancestors in traditional
communities, individuals in modern society appear to have greater
control over continuing relationships. Yet occasionally, because the
dead are mobile and retain spontaneity, they may appear when not
desired. And, as the discussion of haunting in Chapter 9 shows, the
dead can be disturbing if the living lose control over their
manifestations and indeed actions. When this occurs the dead may
exert control over *us*, appearing to people who do not look for nor

want them, being present at the wrong time and in inappropriate places.

Just as death can be read from a variety of sources, the dead too can appear in numerous forms. They need not appear in a whole or embodied fashion. They may, as noted earlier, be experienced only as a smell or a sound. Their presence may jar as they surprise the unwary who recognise them by their handwriting on a page or by the manner in which things are ordered on a shelf. They may transfer physical features of themselves onto other, living bodies. In this way they may be recognised by the colour or style of their hair, by the way in which they walk, the curve of the lip, the intonation in the voice. In these forms they may appear, and be brought to mind, when least expected and sometimes when they are unwelcome.

As the living move on, the dead may not always move with them or fully embrace the widow's new relationships. Like visitations which take over another's body, in dreams the dead may appear in the wrong body, disturbing equilibrium and threatening not only the stability of the living, but the living's perception of the dead.

Conclusion

This chapter has examined the social presence of the dead and challenged a view of society which gives them little weight. As the studies cited indicate, elderly widows may continue to enjoy a social relationship with a biologically dead husband. Indeed, husbands have agency in relation to the woman's life, providing, at various times, companionship, advice, direction and meaning. By enduring as an active agent, the self of the husband is intertwined with the self of the widow. Furthermore, his agency and presence are experienced through her body, not just in the mind but via the senses. As such, her body acts as the site of empowerment for his self. This undermines the notion of the bounded body, inhabited exclusively by the self. It is a continued relationship which threatens the strict binary distinction between life and death. It also transgresses the dominant medical discourse that prescribes giving up relationships with the dead as the recommended panacea for grief. Far from being static, the relationship between the deceased husband and the widow is dynamic, developing in relation to her needs and changing lifestyle. While frequently harmonious and desired, the continued presence of the dead may be unwelcome when experienced by people who would rather locate them within their memories of the past. If, as social scientists, we wish to make sense of the lives of those around us, it is imperative that our model of society is one which takes full account of – rather than excludes – its dead members.

Chapter 9

Ghosts, apparitions and occult phenomena

This chapter continues the previous chapter's discussion of how the self may persist in the absence of the body, whether dying or dead. As we saw, some older adults continue to enjoy a relationship with a deceased spouse or partner and indeed the injunction to 'let go' of the dead, which until recently has underpinned bereavement counselling, is likely to be played down in relation to older people. Arnason states that during training as a counsellor:

> it was implied that the elderly might be excused for continuing their lives as they had lived them with their partners for a life time, but that younger people should...take hold of their lives and try to live them as they want to.
>
> (1998: 139)

If continued bonds between older people and the dead are tolerated, this might reflect nothing more than ageism. As in the case of medical decisions about older people's access to hip replacements or kidney transplants, ageist assumptions may lead to the view that they are not worth 'rehabilitating'. Indeed, if 'eccentric' behaviour is expected of them by younger people, then the 'imagined' presence of the dead within the social world of older adults will, to a certain extent, be expected. The marginalisation of the dead is, in this respect, reinforced through the framework of ageism. While dominant social ideas concerning the elderly might associate advanced age and the domains of the dead, younger adults are expected to maintain distance between themselves and the deceased.

Here we begin to examine the range of beliefs and experiences relating to the dead which characterise Western society. We start with some of the religious frameworks which have retained a dominant position throughout Western history. However, we not only acknowledge the diversity of beliefs and practices among different denominations and officiants; we also recognise the long-standing importance of more marginalised belief systems. Thus, research which explored beliefs and practices surrounding the funeral among Christian clergy, for example, revealed a diversity of contemporary assumptions and strategies in relation to the uncertain fate of the soul of agnostic or even a non-practising Christians (Hockey, 1992). Some ministers spoke of their difficulty in including passages from the liturgy which promised a resurrection to eternal life when the deceased was not evidently a believer. With reference to more marginalised belief systems, Warner highlights 'Counter-Enlightenment' attacks on the cult of reason which developed in the mid-seventeenth century: 'the rebellion against lucidity and rationality pursued metaphysical, Romantic, vitalist, psychic and spiritual knowledge' (1996: 13). However, Warner stresses that even within the Enlightenment tradition, science extended itself beyond what she calls 'purely rational materials'. In the early nineteenth century Anton Mesmer's work provided an 'objective' basis for communication between the living and the dead. Finucane cites Emma Hardinge-Britten's writing on spiritual matters where, in 1881, she describes how Mesmer 'brought the wand of science to bear upon the enchantments of ignorance' (1996: 179). Similarly, the archives of the Society for Psychical Research in the 1920s contain letters from established scientists about spirit photographs and the 'authentic capture of invisible auras and ghosts and presences' (Warner, 1996: 16).

The material which forms the core of this chapter reveals that, while concerns about the dangers of the 'occult' remain deeply embedded within Christian discourse, in the 1990s it continues to harness scientific beliefs and metaphors as a means to explain phenomena which appear to defy 'reason', for example, ghosts, poltergeists and other forms of haunting. We are therefore dealing with belief systems which seek to differentiate themselves from one another, yet paradoxically, share or appropriate one another's repertoires of explanatory principles and classificatory orientations.

Warner argues that occult, or hidden domains encompass 'beliefs, epistemologies, systems that are premised on the existence of an invisible reality that obeys its own rules and exercises significant power over apprehensible and material phenomena' (1996: 69). As discussed in the previous chapter, the concept of 'agency' traditionally adhered to within the social sciences, limits itself to the acts and the effects of human beings who are narrowly defined in empirical terms as 'living'. We have already examined some of the ambiguities which destabilise this apparently unproblematic term, when, for example, we analyse perceptions of the frail elderly, the comatose, the unborn and the stillborn. As these chapters show, 'death', the binary opposite to so slippery a concept as 'life', is, in practice, similarly difficult to define with any precision. This, at least in part, may explain the marginalisation of 'the dead' within empiricist social science. In order to develop debates on these issues, we have drawn upon more recent definitions of agency and examine it, therefore, not as a property of the full-bodied individual, but rather as empowerment at a particular site (see Chapter 8).

Drawing on Keller's (1998) approach to religious belief which proposes that it should be regarded as an embodied, constitutive process rather than a set of ideas which are stored within individual psyches, we here examine the embodied practices involved in 'haunting' and 'exorcism' in a contemporary Western context. In her view the content of such practices needs to be given weight in its own right – rather than being seen simply as a symbolic manifestation of something else. Theoretical orientations which distance themselves from culturally marginalised domains of experience fail to provide an adequate account of that reality. In broad terms, we therefore follow those Counter-Enlightenment thinkers who themselves resisted limited explanatory frameworks. Warner describes them as, 'lay[ing] common stress on the valuable function of fantasy and imagination in the analysis of reality and in the truthful description of human experience and human beings' place in the world' (1996: 13). In his cultural history of ghosts, Finucane adopts a similar, if theoretically more conservative approach to this field when he states:

> [e]ven though ghosts or apparitions may exist only in the minds of their percipients, the fact of that existence is a social and historical reality...as in the case of literary and aesthetic invention, the results cannot be divorced from their social milieu.
>
> (1996: 1)

Apparitions, poltergeists and evil presences

Western eschatology is founded on the differentiation of life from death. Rather than being one stage in a cycle of transitions, Christian death is singled out as life's final punctuation mark. During the history of Western belief, death has been made sense of in terms of a sequence of beliefs, some of which exist in parallel with one another. Pagan assumptions about the dead, for example, carried forward into Christian Europe. The idea that the dead may have a function or role within the lives of the living – 'informing, consoling, admonishing, pursuing' – is a late classical tradition which again recurs throughout the early modern and modern period (Finucane, 1996: 25). By the nineteenth century, however, scepticism and science had so undermined belief in an afterlife, that the one function remaining to the ghost was to satisfy an unresolved yearning for immortality. As Finucane says, 'silent grey ladies who stood at the foot of the bed, and dark nameless figures that floated away without so much as a word' provided a highly satisfactory if unspoken answer to such anxious questioning (ibid.: 212). As noted, the possibility of human continuity in spirit form has been both denigrated as well as researched within the frameworks of positivist science. Christian 'souls' which once journeyed through purgatory in the uncertain hope of resurrection to eternal heavenly life, have, since the Reformation, been consigned to God's immediate judgement and a rapid transition, either to heaven or hell. Rather than post-mortem salvation through the prayers of survivors, deathbed conversion became crucial during the Victorian era if a heavenly afterlife was to be achieved. Walter argues that by the 1920s a hellish afterlife had ceased to be. Neither romantically inclined Victorian spouses and children, nor the relatives of young men eradicated in First World War battles, could contemplate so horrendous a fate for their loved ones (1990: 92–98).

Intrinsic to dualistic models of 'life' defined in relation to 'death' are assumptions about the boundary which both divides and connects these domains. Changing beliefs about its nature and scale impact upon relationships between the living and the dead. Finucane cites Gregory the Great who, in the early Middle Ages said, 'It seems that the spiritual world is moving closer to us, manifesting itself through visions and revelations.' However, as Finucane points out 'the golden age of communication with the dead...was yet to come' (1996: 47). It is during the nineteenth century that a range of methods for achieving 'spectral communication' became popular, for example, rapping, planchette-writing and table tilting. This chapter presents a case study of the work of an Anglican minister who regularly conducts exorcisms for people or within places which are felt to be disturbed in particular ways (Hockey, 1999). We examine aspects of lay and ecclesiastical discourse which situate and define supernatural beings that manifest themselves in embodied and disembodied forms. In doing so, we draw attention to the ways in which dominant Western belief systems differentiate between life as represented by material embodiment and death as represented, variously, by disembodied survival in a spirit world or disembodied immortality through 'great works' or family reminiscences.

When somebody or something which is dead registers its presence, mainstream, positivist models of the corporeal world appear unstable in that their basic epistemological assumptions are open to question. This is not the same as saying that people are frightened of ghosts, since contact with the dead is often sought; for example, by wearing the clothing and appropriating the behaviours of the dead and by consulting with clairvoyants. The public performances of clairvoyants attract audiences of several hundred people, all of whom willingly participate in communication with the dead. The commercialisation of ghost paraphernalia, from fairgrounds to 'olde worlde' ghost tours further attests to their popularity.

When we speak of the dead, therefore, it is perhaps an area which, more than most, reveals the heterogeneity of Western belief systems. On the one hand, the dead can remain almost comfortably at home among the living. For instance, their birthdays are commemorated in local newspapers, their possessions are cherished as reminders of that person, they are evoked in reminiscence and in the naming of their children and grandchildren. For the more famous dead, they may be brought to mind in street names or in public statues. Such practices are significant in that they constitute continuing social identities for the dead, and indeed maintain their social presence. For example, after a death, survivors describe a welcomed sense of the presence of the deceased; reminders of the sight, sound or smell of that person; the evocation of that person through meditation at the graveside; an internalised sense of communion with someone who was very close – a partner or parent; and the seeking out or invocation of someone who is dead via a clairvoyant or through attendance at a spiritualist church.

These are the welcomed dead who feature prominently in Chapters 8 and 10. Finucane points to their persistent spiritual resonances in Christian traditions, where they act as manifestations of the rewarding heavenly life which awaits the true believer. Yet, he cites Huxley's early twentieth century scientific denigration of the evidence provided by seances and spirit mediums as 'the chatter of old women and curates in the nearest cathedral town' (1996: 183). It is the ambiguity of responses to the manifestation of non-ordinary entities and energies which this chapter sets out to capture, an emotional and cognitive dissonance which is evident even in our case study of a single Christian minister. As such, this minister is heir to deep divisions among nineteenth century clerics, some of whom felt a direct antagonism towards the 'alternative creed' of spiritualism, while others participated in the Society for Psychical Research and saw spirit manifestations as corroborations of a Christian promise of immortality (Finucane, 1996: 210–211). This chapter contrasts less welcome experiences of contact with non-worldly beings and phenomena with the manifestations of the dead who seem to co-exist unproblematically among the living. It is the problematic nature of these manifestations and the strategies through which they are managed which we now discuss.

Contemporary Western society can no longer be described as an environment where a continued existence after death is a taken for granted belief. Badham points out that, '[e]ven the journal *Theology* defines life after death as a "fringe belief" in our society' (1989: 209). However, there is a persistent fascination with what is loosely conceptualised as a 'other-worldly domain' at the level of everyday experience and in media representations.

In this and the following chapter we therefore set out to develop a fuller, theoretically informed account of the diversity of beliefs and experiences which surround the relationship between society's living and dead members. Chapter 10 focuses upon systems of embodied communication between these two domains, apparent within the ritualised practices of spiritualists and clairvoyants. The present chapter examines experiences of the 'other' world of the dead from the perspective of a mainstream Christian belief system. This provides an important starting point from which to make sense of the processes through which the dead are marginalised, and yet constantly 'recovered', within Western society.

Matter out of place

Mary Douglas' work (1966) on the classificatory schema, through which societies divide up and thereby assign meaning to their worlds, highlights objects and events, or times and spaces which are not easily accommodated within particular conceptual frameworks. Douglas draws upon Van Gennep's metaphor of society as a house with an internal structure comprised of rooms and corridors separated by boundaries. Passage between these clearly defined spaces is dangerous, just as falling betwixt and between the social categories of one's society is seen as a source of disorder – as matter out of place. Douglas' theoretical perspective offers a means to interpret contemporary perceptions of other-worldly matter or materialisations. Here we examine such experiences as represented through the descriptions of an Anglican minister, believed to have special expertise in dealing with disturbances of a supernatural origin. This case study is based upon an analysis of the minister's address to a women's church group and an extended interview. Of particular interest here is the vocabulary he used when describing hauntings, as well as the attempts he made to map out and systematise a wide domain of disorderly spiritual matter. The minister provided accounts of experiences of such phenomena in cases where he had been requested to intervene or to help people cope. His descriptions, therefore, represent events from his own perspective, but also incorporate reported words from the lay persons involved. The following examples, drawn from the minister's accounts, can be interpreted as texts generated through interactions between a ritual specialist and lay persons seeking to make sense of crises triggered by the 'disorderly' dead.

First, his description of matter which was, quite literally, out of place:

> It was about three o'clock in the morning and their sitting room, they claimed, had been wrecked by...they were upstairs in bed and they said there was absolute chaos, smashing and crashing downstairs. And when they all went downstairs the whole room was in chaos, things had been smashed that were quite precious to them...all sorts of things turned over, the furniture all turned over...chaos.

Another example, again in the minister's own words, which describes the dead appearing in the space of the living:

> Mary said, 'I went into the kitchen, put the sausage rolls in the oven, closed the oven door, turned, there he was stood in the corner, smiling at me [dead ex-husband]. I looked away, looked back...he was still there and slowly he faded. I was absolutely shattered. What's happening to me?'

And similarly: 'Anne said, "I looked up and there, framed in the doorway, was my father and I was absolutely shattered. Nice to see him...but shattered".' And again:

> Maureen said, 'The first time I saw it I screamed the place down...I mean we wouldn't see him for six months and then suddenly for about three weeks he was everywhere, he'd be in the passageway, he'd be by the television, he'd be upstairs, in the kitchen when you were cooking, he'd be everywhere.'

Also a source of alarm are phenomena that defy 'ordinary' experiences of the five senses, in particular the inconsistencies which arise out of occurrences which are perceptible by one sense but not another. In this case something was highly audible yet invisible:

> There was a block of flats, an old house, no other houses nearby...and they'd all been woken up by a man and woman running up and down the stairs screaming at one another and they all turned out to see who was having a row and nobody was, the sound went past them up the stairs and down again and nobody was there...they were terrified.

And a case where something could be detected through smell but not sight:

> A woman rang me up and said, 'Could you come...we've got an evil smell in our house...we've got this evil smell coming...it's all around us...and we've been rehoused three times'...and then the daughter said, 'Here it comes', and the mother said, 'Oh yeah.' And they were coughing and there were tears coming down their faces.

Common to all of these accounts is a tangible sense of unease and very often fear. These sensations are associated with events and encounters which are inconsistent with Western common-sense assumptions regarding persons, objects and domestic spaces. Orderly, everyday routines are disrupted and, not infrequently, people come to doubt their sanity, finding their own derangement easier to grasp than the 'non-sense' of what is apparently unfolding before them. The people described by the minister responded in a variety of ways, with recourse to the police or the Samaritans, their doctors, the social services or the housing department. However they detected these 'material' phenomena – whether through smells, sounds, sights, or the mobilisation of inanimate objects – there is without doubt a powerful embodied process which ensues around such experiences. Indeed these are phenomena which induce a particularly intense bodily experience of panic and alarm, sensations which result in dramatic acts, for example, jumping out of bed in terror and running into the public space of the street, screaming and shouting. People interpret these experiences as disorders which require some kind of re-ordering and thus direct their alarm calls to agencies which represent forces of order and in some cases law. Within this hierarchy of resort, the minister is contacted as a specialist who might be equipped to deal with profoundly anomalous events of a 'spiritual' kind. From the lay perspective, these events 'cannot really be happening', yet they must be taken seriously and eradicated: a strange contradiction, inspired by both a challenge to the normal order of things as well as attempts to deny their possibility.

What are the frameworks of belief through which this kind of occurrence is understood and managed? From the reported descriptions, the perception of a threat to order and to common sense is a powerful element within percipients' experiences. The minister described people's fear that they were going 'mad' and their relief at finding someone who would take them seriously. None the less it is important not to reduce these responses to some kind of cognitive threat – the idea that nothing is more frightening than the unknown or unknowable. Clearly some of the experiences which precipitated the minister's involvement have terrifying properties over and above their failure to fit within the scheme of things – they evoke a strong sense of malevolence or evil. For example, he reports people saying 'We have a terrible sense of menace and threat in the upstairs bedroom'. But in some cases materialisations of the spirit, although lying beyond the limits of 'common sense', could somehow still be accommodated:

> I had a woman who lived in an empty house...a very lonely farmhouse...on her own and said, 'I've got a ghost in my house...but I don't want rid of it. You see I live alone. It's company.' And she saw the old man going down the corridor and 'Oh, there's somebody around', you know. She quite welcomed it...it didn't do her any harm.

Even the woman who 'screamed the place down' when she first saw the old man who was to appear everywhere in her house for weeks said that:

> after a while we got used to it...seems silly but I mean, he never did us any harm...Some nights we'd get the kids off to bed and a bit of peace...and the door would open and one of the kids would look round the door and say, 'Mum...'. I'd say, 'What now!' and they'd say, 'That old man's in our room again'...'Oh, say night, night, God bless, he'll go, he'll go.'

The minister himself, however, represents a case study example of more conventional or institutionalised responses to spirit materialisation. His orientation towards the occurrences he deals with is ambiguous, conceptually as well as emotionally. Certainly, in his work with ghosts and hauntings, he clearly regards himself as charged with the requirement to restore order, to return matter to its rightful place. Ghosts are potentially a problem and he says of one setting: 'it was very badly haunted'. For him this is not to deny the existence of a domain of being outside the material world. Indeed he expresses the view that the dead are closer to us than we are to them. Further, he admits to an 'adolescent' fascination with phantoms, mysteries and what he calls 'weird things'. He says that he is a member of 'the exorcist's tea-party', an event which regularly brings clergy together with psychiatrists, parapsychologists and what he calls 'all sorts of strange people'.

The vocabulary used to express the minister's orientation towards his work suggests a contradiction. The minister is drawn towards that which he sets out to dispel. Thus, for example, when the people in a room he was blessing all pulled away from the walls at the same moment, he reported being 'fascinated' that the room got warmer instantaneously. When asked whether he was ever frightened he said, 'I'm fascinated as to what really is the mystery thing, what is going on here...you're interested so you're not afraid.' He therefore deals with something more than just matter out of place in a problematic sense. Rather, for this minister, a being which materialises, which can be seen, heard, sensed or smelt constitutes the 'other'. It is not part of a natural but a supernatural order. It is someone or something which is both like us and unlike us, a way of knowing oneself and one's limits via the mechanism of difference or opposition. Though the minister sees himself called upon to return the 'other' to a more orderly state of opposition, he does not discount its otherness, nor seek to reduce it to a kind of sameness.

His framework differs markedly from the model which under-pins the work of contemporary spirit mediums. In public perform-ances, the dead are made highly proximate. In one case in the north of England, audience members were asked whether particular relatives were 'this side' or 'the other side' in a manner which suggested a neighbourly closeness between the two domains. Similarly the spirit medium addressed both the audience and their spirit relatives in the same intimate joking language, creating a common, homely focus, for example, through reference to microwaves, DIY and dieting. The minister, however, adheres to a Christian eschatological framework within which there are earthly beings who are 'like us' and spiritual beings who are 'other' in relation to us. In his work as exorcist he deals with an illegitimate intermingling of self and other, and seeks to produce a particular ordering of that relationship. As already pointed out, it is often the nature and scale of the boundary between life and death which are contested, rather than simply the question of post-mortem survival. While the minister draws on religious authority to access, patrol and maintain a distinctive life:death boundary, the stage medium locates himself within a spiritualist tradition of belief and practice to produce an intimate, connecting link between these two domains. While the homeliness of the 'afterlife' he produces represented an important point of identification for his audience, it is precisely the mundanity of visions of this kind which so ruffled the scientist, Huxley, who ironically claimed that spiritualism provided a useful disincentive to suicide: 'Better live a crossing-sweeper than die and be made to talk twaddle by a "medium" hired at a guinea a seance' (Finucane, 1996: 184).

Agent of order

As noted, in the search for a means to control disturbing appearances of the dead, people will phone the police or the Samaritans. Yet a decision is often made that such events require the intervention of a minister of the church rather than a member of a legal or medical institution. This may not be an easy decision to make and evidence is often weighed up carefully. For instance, soil experts, plumbers, sanitary people and local counsellors may be called in before recourse is finally made to a minister of the church. Within the sociology of deviance, labelling theory suggests that crime has no absolute existence but represents the product of a set of interpretations made by, among others, members of the criminal justice system (Becker, 1963). In the case of the 'deviant' occurrences which the minister responds to, certain materialisations or noises have come to be constituted, at least tentatively, as supernatural. As the minister stated:

> The police ring me up and say, 'We've got a family out in the street. We think it's more your department. Could you deal with it?' or 'Do you mind if you deal with it? I think it's more your thing anyway.'

Some preliminary interpretation has therefore been made. Though neither the troubled individuals, nor the representatives of the agency they contact may adhere to any religious belief, it is to the Church which they turn in the face of events which fall beyond the boundaries of the human phenomenological world. While the data presented do not show how the individuals, the police or the Samaritans actually 'produce' the ghost or the phantom, the minister himself illuminated the next stage in that process, detailing his thoughts and practices when summoned by an agency or individual. These include entering each situation from a position of scepticism and then drawing on a whole range of explanatory frameworks before taking action. None the less, as argued at the beginning of this chapter, we are not approaching this material from a theoretical perspective which locates 'belief' as something internal to the practitioner or officiant. Rather, we make sense of his response by viewing it as an embodied set of practices through which the 'materialisation of the spirit' is brought into being. Indeed, as the minister's testimony indicates, this area of his professional life involves dramatic experiences of his own body – even though he claims never to have 'seen' a ghost.

From science to Scooby-Doo

The minister argued that 'there are lot of phenomena which science has not yet coped with in any generation'. And he went on to describe water jetting out of living room walls, objects moving through brick walls, and individuals who can will objects to move. However, rather than religious language, his discussion of other-worldly phenomena is couched in the terminology of science and technology. He thus echoes the nineteenth century link between spiritualism and science when, for example, an 1884 issue of the spiritualist monthly *Spiritual Record* claimed that it treated 'the whole subject of Spiritual manifestations exactly as it would any branch of Science' (cited in Oppenheim, 1985). Oppenheim describes the scientific method as 'hailed, almost reverently' during this period, a self-evidently powerful way of establishing the validity of spiritualism (ibid.: 199). A century later a minister still accounts for his bodily experiences of the spirit world in the language of the natural sciences and technology. For example, he describes 'bolts of electricity' moving through him; he accounts for the human ability to see spirits in terms of 'inner instincts' and having 'those genes that see ghosts'; he uses the term 'the zigzags' to conjure up what he describes as 'an electricky feeling' precipitated by unseen presences; he refers to 'stressed energy', 'three-dimensional holograms', 'tape-recordings', 'photographs' and 'videos' to account for the re-appearance of violent or tragic events from the past. While the minister's interest in scientific explanations for spiritual phenomena is serious, his language, arguably, is a metaphorical strategy rather than a systematic attempt to rationalise the irrational. It is his use of the language of science and technology which signals the 'otherness' of the phenomena in question. Though he envisages a transformed science which might one day encompass supernatural phenomena, science is currently unable to 'cope' with them. Science does, however, provide a cultural resource, used when accounting for the 'otherness' of the supernatural.

This possibility arises from the way in which the natural sciences are represented, at least in the popular imagination, as objective or neutral. While social scientists have challenged this view, at an everyday level, science is still seen as a domain which stands outside culture, as value-free knowledge, based upon measurement, testing and proof. Thus the instruments of science and technology, such as the watch or the camera, cannot lie. As machines they are above the vagaries of human emotion. If they fail to provide a measurement of time or an image of the material world, then the fault is seen as mechanical rather than one of human error. Science therefore appears to stand outside the flux of unpredictable human action. It occupies a different realm by virtue of its sources in objectivity and measurement. As such, it provides an apt source of metaphors through which to represent a similarly distanced domain, the world of ghosts and hauntings. In relation to this rhetorical elision of the domains of the science and the supernatural, we can note Emma Hardinge-Britten's earlier, parallel use of magical imagery – 'the wand of science' – to promote Anton Mesmer's status as a scientist of the spiritual world (Finucane, 1996: 179). Indeed, the mysterious, even arcane properties of science and technology, lend additional resonance as a rhetorical resource.

Thus, in addition to its aspirations to value-free objectivity, science stands apart from the everyday world by virtue of its magical or fantastical properties. For example, although fire-making by rubbing sticks together is an unpredictable business when compared with flicking an electric switch, we do have a greater sense for what is happening – we grasp the sticks, feel the warmth being generated and see the first sparks. But how much do we understand about the link between our finger and the heat in an element when we flick a switch? The connection has a magical quality. If it breaks we cannot fix it. If we handle it incorrectly it will kill us.

It can therefore be argued that in representing the otherness of supernatural phenomena through the extra-ordinariness of science and technology, the minister sets it apart and so underscores its difference. Listening to him we learn that it lies outside the realms of human society and beyond the realm of mundane understanding – doubly fantastical. Additionally, in the language which he uses the power of scientific metaphors is enhanced by a set of different images from other non-ordinary domains, that is, the fields of imagination or play. For example, the superhuman qualities of a cartoon character, a toy or ventriloquist's dummy are drawn upon. In one particularly powerful 'material' experience, the minister felt an electrical shock enter his body and then pass down the line of family members beside him. He claims:

> my knees shot together and my elbows shot together and head whiplashed back – pow! – like this, and I got sort of...not a cricked neck but a headache, a sort of top headache for about twenty minutes afterwards from this whiplash, from all the sort of crumple. And they said I shrivelled...

Accounting for a violent and inexplicable attack on his body, he turns to cartoon imagery to describe the experience: 'Some entity...coming through the three of us...doing a kind of Scooby-Doo'. Similarly, he described a meeting with a medium who had punctuated his conversation with asides to a spirit, or as the minister put it, had 'a kind of Emu on his shoulder'. Via the playful image of Rod Hull's persistently aggressive dummy, the minister metaphorically debunks the supposed spirit while hinting at its malevolent power to attach itself to the living. He also uses a 'stagey' humour to lend a farcical nature to the hauntings he has attended: 'You go up there and you go "Ooh-er!" because the family say, "Oh, by the way, there's no light in that bedroom"; You open the door and look into blackness but you've heard footsteps coming.' Pantomime dialogue between audience and comic character is hinted at when he says:

> I've never seen a ghost. I've been there when people have said, 'It's behind you!', you know...and run out!...Quite often I'll be blessing a house and I get to the landing, and as I get there they say, 'It's there', and I say, 'Where?' They say, 'In the corner!' I say, 'Which corner?' They say, 'Left one!' and they're off downstairs...and then I go and bless the left one and there's nothing there as far as I'm concerned.

However, on numerous occasions he has the intensely physical sensation of the 'zigzags', which indicates to him an unseen presence in the room. Describing this bodily experience, he refers to Peter Sellers' Inspector Clouseau who would have his servant jump out at him to teach him to respond to sudden attacks. In a description of his first high-profile exorcism, which was conducted on a trawler which would only go round in circles, he referred to a TV advert where comic Roman oarsmen sweat away, rowing in a circular motion. He also cited a lay reader who was on board and quipped, 'I can't swim. I'm on a boat which is haunted and I can't swim' and the jokey media headlines which later reported the event: 'Holy Mackerel', 'In the Name of Cod' and 'Holy Water Relaunches Ship'.

In his retrospective reflection on these cases, the minister claimed: 'when you're in the middle of it you just cannot believe what you're experiencing because things don't normally go through brick walls'. In his attempts to explain these events, he draws on domains which do not belong to the common-sense, material world, whether they be the 'magical' sphere of science, or the make-believe arena of imaginary creatures or of farce. As a result we develop a sense of the ambiguous position of the materialised spirit, betwixt and between the serious yet safe categories of the known world. 'Flesh' and 'self', normally separable at death within both religious as well as medical frameworks, begin to obtrude upon one another. Via the mixed metaphors of fantasy, danger and play an other world of ghosts and hauntings is conjured into its separate space – and the coherence of materialist world views is allowed to stand firm.

Re-positioning the other

As shown in the material already presented, the capacity of ghosts and hauntings to both demand yet persistently elude an explanation fascinates the minister. As a former member of the local Magic Circle, he relishes a mystery. However, as a minister of the church, his role is, quite literally, to minister to the needs of his parishioners and others. Therefore, in parallel with the mixing of fantastical or playful metaphors, the minister also draws upon a second, rather different range of mutually reinforcing images. These are more closely aligned with issues of power and control.

The minister's starting point is the authority of the Church of England. He invokes a privileged access to the sacred, echoing the Right Reverend Brooke Foss Westcott, Bishop of Durham, who, in 1893, said:

> It appears to me that in this, as in all spiritual questions, Holy Scripture is our supreme guide...I cannot, therefore, but regard every voluntary approach to beings such as those who are supposed to hold communication with men through mediums as unlawful and perilous.
>
> (Oppenheim, 1985)

Many of the phenomena which the minister is called out to deal with are, in his view, the result of what he calls 'the occult explosion', the aftermath of the 1951 repeal of the Witchcraft Act which made it legal to conduct seances with *ouija* boards, to consult tarot cards and to visit mediums. In seeking illegitimate access to the sacred, by 'dabbling in the occult', the minister believed that individuals might open channels which could be appropriated by evil spirits rather than the 'good' dead. If they stumble upon a personal aptitude for channelling useful or comforting information from the dead towards the living, this would later be revealed as a misleading illusion. In time, an evil spirit will colonise this channel and begin to communicate mischievous or distressing information, so disrupting peaceful lives and trusting relationships.

The metaphors through which the minister accounted for his legitimate access to the sacred draw analogies between his own role and those of experts in the institutions of medicine and law. As Turner (1987) notes, religion, medicine and law have only recently been differentiated from one another through the creation of separate professional organisations. Such is their persistent relationship in the governing of the soul, the body and the state, that an appeal to one in turn connotes the other two. Thus, when called out in the early hours of the morning, the minister says that 'I used to jump into the car and zoom off, sort of ecclesiastical policewise.' Extending the metaphor, he describes the 'detective work' which his 'cases' involve – finding evidence which establishes the truth behind what people are telling him, discovering who the witnesses were and whether they are reliable, and whether the testimonies of different witnesses are consistent. When dealing with severe poltergeist activity, the minister described his internal dialogue as follows:

> There's five things on that mantlepiece. I'm looking at them. I know they're there. I've got them in my mind and about twenty minutes later one of the family would say, 'Dog orna-ment's gone again'. And I'd look and it had gone and…you look round…all doors and windows are closed…and you think, 'Now, come on,…now, if while I was talking to mother, hus-band put it in his pocket…but surely I would have seen it as we're all in this close proximity'…and I think, 'Well, if one is doing it and playing tricks, they must all be in on it because

the others must have seen it happening, so why are they doing it?'

Albeit in the metaphorical role of sleuth, the minister also used medical imagery which evokes both the individual physician and the public health doctor. Thus the process of healing is a predominant feature in his interview material. Again, the metaphor is extended when he describes an exorcism, 'it works in a funny sort of way and my argument is, if the cure works then your diagnosis must be somewhere near the truth'. And:

> Sometimes you bless a place and it works, everything's alright after that and you think, 'Well, I don't know what we've dealt with there.' And some doctors will say 'Don't know what those spots were but the cream worked, fair enough, you know.' So, you're somewhere near the diagnosis. You're not bang on perhaps but you've applied the cure for that particular problem and it's worked, so whatever.

Public health imagery is also evident when he represents evil via the concepts of contagion, hygiene and public sanitation. It is something which 'sort of infests places' where Satan has been worshipped or where individuals have 'dabbled in the occult'. As a result 'weird things' can happen, by contagion, to innocent people who stray into certain parts of the woods or particular buildings.

In all of this, the minister acknowledges the similarity and indeed overlap between his work and that of psychiatrists. Playing a literal rather than metaphorical role in his account, these experts also seek to heal, cure or dispel disorder, the appropriate division of labour not always being apparent. Thus individuals who approach the minister often fear for their own sanity – 'Am I heading for a nervous breakdown, as my husband says, or is my house haunted?' He in turn addresses the same question:

> Somebody comes for laying on of hands and starts shaking and screaming and speaking in a foreign language...you think is this possession or is this person schizophrenic...let's get somebody else...and see if we can get some medical reports on him.

And finally the agents of order themselves struggle to map their remedies onto disorderly experience. The minister described 'a hilarious situation where the psychiatrist was saying, "We think he's possessed!" and I'm saying, "No, he isn't!"...you'd expect it the other way round...throwing him backwards and forwards.'

Systems of classification are therefore under threat at both their external and internal boundaries. In a broad sense, it can be difficult to label the matter which is out of place. By definition, it eludes categorisation. It might be 'madness', 'trickery', 'bad plumbing' or a 'ghost'. Once it has been assigned to a broad class of disorder, it is then subject to further classificatory processes. This can be seen as an important dimension of returning the matter to its rightful place, of wielding expert power. It is a different process to that which produced its 'otherness', one which plays on the domains of fantasy and magic.

When the minister addressed the church women's group on the theme of 'Ghosts and God', his aim was to instruct rather than entertain. As a man of the church he structured his talk around five categories of 'occult disturbance'; two- or three-dimensional apparitions of the dead; physical hauntings which involve the movement of objects, temperature changes and smells; poltergeist disturbances focused on a particular individual; evil presences; and malevolent forecasts produced through occult practices. Thus, that which can pass through walls and play games with the rules of physics, is here subjected to internal ordering via the imposition of a culturally specific classificatory system. The minister had printed a leaflet with the aim of introducing new clergy to the field of exorcism and, as well as the five categories, it also itemised the six tasks of dealing with such phenomena. Novice exorcists are advised to question every aspect of the situation – what is happening, when, where, to whom, why and how can I help? Rather than the production of otherness, the minister in his guise of instructor offers a mode of control which situates a haunting in relation to the spatial and temporal co-ordinates of everyday life.

Alive and 'British'

Thus far we have emphasised the epistemological dilemmas which arise when spirits materialise. However, this is not to reduce their power to a purely cognitive or classificatory problem. Rather, it is to highlight the cultural marginalisation of phenomena of this kind, to question their relegation to the more obscure class marks of a library's cataloguing system. Here we concur with Paul Badham

(1989) that, however central a belief in immortality might be to a system of religious belief, the Western dead have been ousted from their space within the cultural imaginary. Though at a conceptual level they remain as the other half of the binary pair, the living and the dead, they are the shadow selves of the living, pressed into service merely as a way of delimiting the time and space of human existence.

This kind of dualism is apparent in the data presented in this chapter. It pervades both the construction of 'otherness' via scientific and playful imagery, as well as the re-positioning or re-ordering of the other via the metaphors of society's key institutions of control. In addition, a nationality-based opposition between the 'British' and 'foreigners' was introduced by the minister as a way of affirming the existence of spirit phenomena as a category of otherness which merited his serious attention. Thus, throughout an extended interview, he made repeated reference to 'sensible people', to 'objective proof', to the need to 'keep your feet on the floor'. It is out of the common-sense testimony of ordinary people that he conjures the phenomena he deals with. Since he is unable to see ghosts for himself, it is the testimony of 'sensible people' which validates and gives substance to the matter in hand. And it is precisely the down-to-earth qualities of witnesses such as farmers and miners which he places in opposition to the unpredictable, noisy and insubstantial beings who trespass among the living. Their materialisations are markers of disordered lives and they emerge in these accounts as the confused victims of tragic accidents, suicides or restless souls. By contrast, those whose testimonies give substance to such phenomena share a set of common characteristics, down-to-earth people who are epitomised in the concept of Britishness.

Britishness is also central to the re-positioning of the other at a safe distance from the living. The minister found that matter out of place almost always meant 'matters getting out of hand'. People run out into the street in terror after a haunting and most of his accounts made reference to the need to calm people down. This he achieves via what he calls 'the usual British thing, make a cup of tea'. For example, the minister reports that when an invisible shrieking couple finally ceased running up and down the stairwell of the old block of flats and the front door swung open and then slammed shut, he deflated its power to inspire horror amongst the other occupants as follows:

> I find myself saying…true Englishman…'Well, whatever it was, it's gone!' And they're all standing on the stairs roaring with laughter and went happily to bed. And I thought after this…how British…you know, something happens and you just laughed at it.

Thus, while the minister might empower himself via images of religious authority and professional expertise when commanding a spirit to leave a house, he also undermines the disruptive power of that entity via his own 'Britishness'. As he said:

> I'm British, which is a help…the British have this ability not to believe what is happening. An American commentator said the best people to have with you in a crisis are the British. The difficulty is persuading the British that there is a crisis and there's an element of that in me.

When the dead enter the space of the living, when they reclaim the materiality of the body which has been disposed of, when families rush screaming into the street in the small hours of the morning and when domestic technology 'goes berserk', the double dualisms of the living and the dead, the phlegmatic British and the excitable Foreigner become destabilised. The minister is in part an agent of order attempting to reconstruct a system in crisis. However, in his refusal to limit himself to metaphors of control, we argue that he is also providing an alternative set of interpretations which indeed allow the dead to be positioned as close at hand, which provide them with an identity and a foothold within everyday life.

It is the place of the dead within the cycle of everyday life which we turn to in Chapter 10. One of Finucane's core arguments is that post-eighteenth century ghosts were positioned within a more remote society. Not that they became less accessible or more infrequent in their appearances. Rather, 'the dead progressively withdrew from direct involvement in familial affairs, becoming at the same time almost exclusively symbols or tokens of immortality for their percipients' (1996: 222). Perceptions of these more anonymous or estranged spirits were, he argues, entirely to be expected in a society where family and community ties were weakening. He contrasts them with what were regarded as more actively communicative spirits of the sixteenth and seventeenth centuries, exemplified in the ghost of Hamlet's father who clearly retained a strong interest in family affairs. Not only does he ensure the reversal of his murdering brother's succession to the throne of Denmark; he also precipitates the deaths of almost every member of the cast. Clearly this was a ghost which exercised a powerfully felt agency.

The logic of Finucane's argument, which contrasts different historical examples, assumes the disappearance of an earlier model of the family and so overlooks the persistence of family and interpersonal ties, albeit in less traditional forms. Crucial to the practices of the Christian minister is a 'detective' role which, in many cases, uncovers strong familial motivations and attachments. Divorced husbands, lonely grandads and worried mothers-in-law are prominent among the examples he describes. After his visit to one woman and her daughter dogged by an evil smell, he 'probed around a bit' and found that there had been another daughter who was disabled and lived in residential care. She had died as a result of scalding in boiling hot bath water. Clearly the minister made a strong familial connection: 'and I thought, what's the smell of somebody…check up whether there's a particular smell for that…'. Similarly, in the case of the furniture violently thrown around in the small hours of the morning, he eventually tracked down the daughter of a woman who had previously lived in the house. He asked her whether there was any reason why her mother might want to get in touch with her living relatives. She told him that there were 'things happening in the family she would not have really…'. In light of the chaos unleashed in her former home, the daughter's reported remark is significant: 'if my mother couldn't get to me she would go berserk'. The woman's dead mother was described as someone determined to retain her grip on family affairs.

Conclusion

We therefore suggest that Finucane's account skirts an informal domain of belief and practice associated with intra-familial relationships which continue to link the living and the dead. As noted, these are evident to an extent in the material provided by the Christian minister. In addition, these are increasingly prominent in the case of the stage mediums. In the case referred to earlier, many members of one medium's audience had arrived in large family groups. When spirits 'made contact' via the medium, families worked collectively to identify their relative from the information transmitted to them. Once channels were opened into the 'other side', dead family members were perceived to 'queue up' or even 'jostle' with one another to get a hearing. Their messages conveyed the familiar tone of family interactions: approval for a change of hairstyle; encouragement to continue dieting; amusement about a daughter who had got something stuck to the sole of her shoe when out for a walk. In Chapter 10 this kind of family interaction is demonstrated with even greater intensity. At times of life crisis and family upheaval it is precisely the dead who are consulted by the living via the clairvoyant. Though Finucane cites Keith Thomas' observation that interpersonal problems are now solved through alternative means, whether technological or political (1996: 223), our data suggest that the dead are in no sense exiled. On the contrary, contact with them is often valued and their interventions are seen to carry serious repercussions. If we take empowerment at a particular site as a definition of agency, then the restriction of its theoretical scope to studies of the living renders even more invisible those members of society whose 'embodiment' may be either achieved through the body of another, or manifested in a more fluid and creative form. In the data presented in this chapter we find evidence of inter-subjective selves which not only encompass the embodied living but also incorporate the disembodied dead.

Chapter 10

Mediating the dead

Spiritualists and clairvoyants

In Wise's 1963 film *The Haunting*, a group of ghost hunters, led by an anthropologist, visit a house in order to analyse the 'disturbances' within its walls. The central visual space of this film is occupied by a disembodied presence which makes its self known primarily through written messages and increasingly violent sounds which manifest throughout the house. These spirit communications are centred on one particular female character, a woman who is represented as 'unstable' and 'vulnerable', who rapidly becomes known as the object of the spirit's desires. The spirit will not rest until it has possessed the woman and thus the film represents the process through which one woman is brought to her death by a powerful disembodied agent. Similarly, in Hitchcock's 1940 version of *Rebecca*, the film's narrative, dialogue and visual space are dominated by the presence of the deceased Mrs Rebecca de Winter. Even after her death, Rebecca's desires, routines, and intentions continue to organise the household spaces of Manderley, as well as the relationships which unfold within them. This is orchestrated mainly through the efforts of Mrs Danvers, Rebecca's housekeeper, who preserves Rebecca's possessions and treasures the memory of the beautiful and powerful woman.

Such dramatic representations of disembodied agency which breach the boundaries of life and death, natural and supernatural, are embedded in Western popular fiction and fantasy. Yet they connect in significant ways with the more mundane experiences of women and men who continue to feel the presence of lost loved ones and who communicate, in a variety of ways, with the deceased (see Chapter 8). The present chapter is concerned with social practices which mediate the living and the dead as well as ritualised encounters, both historical and contemporary, which draw the embodied living and the dead into meaningful relationships.

The previous chapters' focus on the construction of social identity via relationships between the living and the dead is here developed in an examination of the work of spiritualist and 'magical' practitioners such as clairvoyants. Here we challenge the assumed fixity of the boundaries which delineate the tangible or 'empirically observable' domains of the living and the 'invisible' and therefore marginalised spheres of the departed. We find that despite the dominance of theories of secularisation and rationalisation in Western societies, there are continuities in magical belief, and a persistent concern with the spiritual, the erotic and the uncontrollable aspects of self and society. Such continuities within contemporary society provide the framework within which we examine conceptions of the living body in relation to manifestations of the deceased. Ritualised encounters, within spiritualist churches or during clairvoyants' consultations, can be crucial in the reconstitution of self and identity at points of crisis such as death. Rather than the cadaver, it is the living body of the medium or the spiritualist church member, the clairvoyant or her client which becomes a resource through which the dead, in spirit form, find a continued social presence.

Relationships between the living and the dead, as well as the techniques and rituals employed in the mediation of these domains, should be understood in the context of Western religious and epistemological frameworks. Thomas demonstrates the prevalence of a wide domain of interconnected magical beliefs in sixteenth century England, including witchcraft, astrology, palmistry and physiognomy (1971: 755). There was little distinction between the established Catholic Church and belief in magical powers until the Protestant Reformation, during which the Church attempted to eradicate popular magical practices. Processes of secularisation redefined the social significance of religious belief and practice. From a sociological perspective, Bruce defines secularisation in terms of 'the decline of popular involvement with churches; the decline in scope and influence of religious institutions; and the decline in the popularity and impact of religious beliefs' (1996: 26). These transformations were related to complex factors, unfolding from the seventeenth century onwards: increasing social fragmentation and breakdown of community; the freeing of economic production from influence by the church; economic growth and specialisation; and increasing rationalisation which underpinned developments in science and technology (ibid.: 51).

Alongside this emphasis on secularisation, cultural historians have attempted to recover the significance of marginalised belief systems. For instance, Warner argues that European magical beliefs and rituals have persisted despite the Enlightenment with its emphasis on reason and rationality. But she points out that these rich Western traditions have been denied, and furthermore, that the 'uses of magic and fantasy have often been ascribed to the Other, to the Stranger, who is consequently characterised as primitive, barbaric, even inhuman' (Warner, 1996: 13).

The association of magical belief with non-Western 'others' is reflected in anthropological studies at the level of ethnographic focus and theoretical elaboration. While earlier ethnographic work on magic was conducted in non-Western societies, (for example, Evans-Pritchard's on the Azande [1937]), there is continued anthropological debate surrounding 'transcultural conceptualisations' such as 'supernatural' and 'belief' (Levy et al., 1996: 13).

In a cross-cultural analysis of spirits, Levy et al. point out that in English terminology, 'spiritual' refers to 'non-materiality', but propose that this is not universal in that some societies identify spirits with varying degrees of corporeality. 'They [spirits] are not, indeed, immaterial, but they are certainly less grossly material than the bodies of physical objects; and it is this subtler mode of corporeal existence that may be called "spiritual" in an ethnological sense' (Lowie, 1970: 99–100, cited in Levy et al., 1996: 12). Furthermore, while spirits are typically located at the margins of a given social world, they are tangible in that 'people know they exist through the sensory warrant of their own experience' (ibid.: 15). The direct relationship between spirits and embodied experience is demonstrated most powerfully in the process of possession. 'Bodies provide the vehicle by means of which spirits can be held in focus, as it were, through which they can be sustained in steady communication, and from which they can be expected to speak' (Lambek, 1996: 240). This, in turn, impinges upon the ways in which social identity is conceived,

> [w]hen a body is taken over in full possession the inhabited self is transformed and the body becomes the identified place where two or more fully formed selves contend – selves with

their own voices, intentions and different kinds of social skills.

(Levy et al., 1996: 18)

The epistemological implications of possession are also significant in that a possessed person is often able to 'reveal socially suppressed material' based upon knowledge which is seen as 'intuitively true, but coming from beyond the overtly tolerable, discussible and often thinkable knowledge of family or culture' (ibid.: 19). Thus, since spirits 'are associated with hidden meanings because they represent suppressed modes of knowing' (ibid.: 19), an analysis of embodied communication with spirits raises key questions with regard to experiential and embodied sources of knowledge, together with their positioning in relation to dominant epistemologies. Furthermore, Tiryakian argues, in relation to Western forms of the occult, that, '[k]nowledge of the invisible is power to transform the visible. It is awesome, fascinating, dangerous knowledge. It is the knowledge of the Magus, whether he be socially designated as a magician, a priest, a scientist, or a charismatic leader' (1974a: 10).

The forms of embodiment produced within systems of religious belief and practice have recently begun to receive more attention. For instance, Mellor and Shilling explore religion as an important factor in the formation of connections between embodiment and sociality. They are concerned with longer-term transformations as well as continuities in modes of embodiment, which they examine in religious and cultural context from the medieval period onwards (1997: 3–4). They identify three main 're-formations' of the body: first, the 'medieval body', characterised by its 'sensuous immersion in the supernatural'; second, the 'Protestant body' which forms a site of control, order and discipline; third, the 'baroque modern body' which is 'Janus-faced' in that it exhibits chronic reflexivity and seeks experts' advice but is, at the same time, associated with 'uncertainty', 'fragmentation' and the 'resurgence of irrational sensuality' (ibid.: 12). Mellor and Shilling suggest that such reformations of the body are not complete or 'uni-dimensional'. For instance, they argue that in contemporary Western societies people 'seek opportunities to reconsecrate the profane' in the search of an immediacy of experience, emotion and passion associated with medieval bodies. This is reflected in the 'renewed interest in fate, destiny, the stars, magic, tarot, nature, cults and games of chance' (ibid.: 26). And furthermore:

[m]odern bodies may conduct 'whispered conversations' with
the dead, for example, but we must not be surprised if baroque
modern bodies [re]turn to seances or other magical forms of
communication, or display an increasing concern with other-
worldly or extra-terrestrial phenomena.

(ibid.: 26)

Mellor and Shilling suggest that the reinvention of such traditions
might be explained in terms of nostalgia and the sense of alienation
from the body generated within highly rationalised environments.

In the context of sociological studies in France it is observed that
'[s]tripped of legitimacy, astrology in the eighteenth and nineteenth
centuries (along with alchemy, palmistry, clairvoyance and
telepathy) encountered both legal and sociocultural repression'.
Consequently, during this period astrology took two forms. On the
one hand, it was diffused and coded as superstitious folk belief. On
the other hand, it took on a clandestine aspect as occultist astrology
in the doctrinal teachings of secret societies and esoteric sects
(Fischler, 1974). With regard to contemporary Western societies,
sociologists highlight the difficulty in defining the occult in that it
is deployed in different ways by various interest groups which tends
to shift its meanings over time:

it is a residual category, a wastebasket, for knowledge claims
that are deviant in some way, that do not fit the established
claims of science or religion. And once such a knowledge claim
gains acceptance within establishment science or religion, it
loses its status as an occultism.

(Truzzi, 1974: 245)

There is, however, a recognition that, in the later twentieth century,
there is an

'occult revival' which is embedded in cultural change and the
dynamics of modernisation and linked to a loss of confidence in
established symbols and cognitive models of reality, in the
exhaustion of institutionalised collective symbols of identity.

(Tiryakian, 1974b: 245)

Despite these sociological claims, there have been relatively few anthropological studies which analyse late twentieth century spirituality and magic in Britain, with the important exceptions of Skultans' (1974) study of spiritualism and mediums in South Wales, Luhrmann's (1989) work on witchcraft and magical practices in London and Okely's (1996) account of fortune-telling in the context of the formation of gypsy identity in England. But in general, within anthropology, the study of contemporary clairvoyant practices remains a marginalised field. Clairvoyants have somehow slipped through the classificatory net and remain largely unexplored. The positioning of clairvoyants at the margins of anthropology is perhaps an unquestioned reflection of local perceptions and wider public debates. Clairvoyants are often regarded with suspicion and sceptical reserve while dominant views in the media represent clairvoyants in terms of theatrical entertainment – they are exploited as a commercial resource or denigrated as tricksters.

This chapter examines these contemporary beliefs and ritual practices from a different perspective to explore embodiment and social identity as constituted through mediumship and clairvoyance. While spiritualists might encounter spirits through the powerful enactment of possession, clairvoyants establish different connections with the deceased, ranging from sustained dialogue in the same ritual space to brief sightings in 'mental' pictures and tarot cards. While attending to the locally perceived and socially organised differences between spiritualists and clairvoyants, we support Lambek's claim that 'no rigidly formulated boundary exists between one religious system and another' (Lambek, 1996: 242). Similarly, Jorgensen and Jorgensen assert that 'a functional distinction between "magic" and "religion" is almost impossible to sustain empirically; and it certainly is not useful, except in the most *ad hoc* and *a priori* fashion, to differentiate among socially marginal beliefs and groups' (1982: 387). They state this with regard to contemporary occult practices, yet their statement echoes what Thomas has argued with regard to the interdependency of popular magical belief and the pre-Reformation church in England (Thomas, 1971). In this historical context the separation of these domains was attempted through the reforming policies of the Protestant Church in efforts to extend control over spiritual belief and practice.

The continuity between systems of belief and ritual practice constitutes one area of complexity, while others emerge when we acknowledge the different perceptions of spiritual activity which co-exist within the same system. As Lambek points out, spirits are encountered in different ways: 'They may be sharply defined, their voices clear and their presence highly framed, or they may retreat to the fuzzy margins or fleeting glimpses, ephemeral presence, inarticulate speech' (1996: 245). This chapter begins with a discussion of embodiment, conceptions of self and disembodied agency based on Skultans' detailed ethnographic study of spiritual-ists in South Wales (1974). It then moves on to explore the ways in which clairvoyants' practices invoke images and voices of the dead. Here we find clairvoyants using a variety of tools and techniques that establish connections of varying intensity with spirits. At the centre of both forms of ritual practice is the living body through which the dead are recovered and interpreted as active social agents.

Embodied traces of the dead

With reference to nineteenth century England, Beer explores 'a different imagining of the invisible' (1996: 86). She quotes John Henry Newman who, in 1843, proposed that, '[t]he world of spirits, then, though unseen, is present; present, not future, not distant' (ibid.: 87). Spiritualist interpretations emphasised that spirit 'emanations take on physical form and lost presences may be materially evoked' (Beer, 1996: 87). This fascination with the invisible is further evidenced in the use of photographic plates in the nineteenth century to capture the presence of spirit forms (see Warner, 1996). An intersection of technological and spiritualist discourses appears, given the parallels between this photographic development and the process by which mediums receive an 'impression' of words or thoughts from spirits (Skultans, 1974). Furthermore, contemporary clairvoyants use photographs in the mediation of the living and the dead. Here we are concerned with the ways in which the living body, in particular ritualised contexts, yields tangible traces of the departed and enters into a process of communication through which the invisible domains of the dead are rendered visible.

Skultans' work, *Intimacy and Ritual* (1974), is a detailed ethno-graphic study which describes the complex dynamics between earthly and spiritual domains. She focused on a group of approxi-mately 400 spiritualists, 80 per cent of whom were women, and pays particular attention to the ways in which spiritualist activity and ritual influenced perceptions of gender roles. In a social context in which women experienced difficulties within marriage and with the 'traditional' roles expected of them, spiritualist rituals provided a forum in which conflicts, frustrations and difficulties were identified and managed. Of particular interest here are Skultans' ethnographic examples which reveal the conceptions of the body, self and identity which were reinforced through ritualised communication with the departed. The following discussion of relationships between embodiment and disembodied agency is based on Skultans' ethnographic accounts.

Her work stresses the importance of 'individual inspiration' in the shaping of local religious belief and practice rather than the written tradition of official spiritualist doctrine (1974: 3). Thus different mediums would lead church meetings and contribute to the dissemination of spiritualist ideas. For example, she notes the dramatic sermon of one woman in March 1969 which contemplated the nature of life and death: 'we are bruised and hurt in the birth pangs of self-realisation,...in death our true selves emerge', and 'after death we become what we truly are now' (ibid.: 15–16). At the same time there are tensions inherent within spiritualist doctrine in that there is a communally sanctioned search for personal salvation but at the same time 'encounters with spirit offer and tempt towards a search for personal power' (ibid.: 61). A deep concern with the spirit world articulates a desire for spiritual development and also provides a channel through which power and authority is acquired and contested (see also Chapter 9).

Skultans notes of the spiritualist group with whom she worked, that there was a general acceptance that a spirit world existed and could be accessed by a variety of means. Within their belief system, the spirit world is organised into a hierarchy in which the lower ranks of spirits are mutually interdependent and regularly communicate with human beings. Immediately after death, spirits remain attached to their earthly conditions and require the help of mediums to release them. This is particularly the case with spirits who died violently or painfully. Before ascending into the higher realms of the spirit world, spirits would return to provide advice and help for the living, while some would actively inflict sickness (ibid.: 33–34). Furthermore, Skultans points out that beliefs about the spirit world and mediumship are not marginal in relation to established churches in that they were 'formerly expressed within orthodox Christian thought' (ibid.: 7). While spiritualists maintain a commitment to the ideology that everyone has 'psychic power in a latent if not fully developed form' (ibid.: 3), communication with spirit is carefully managed and usually undertaken by experienced mediums. In organised circles or wider church meetings, contact with the other world is achieved through 'possession', 'impression' and 'message giving'.

In the context of the spiritualist meetings, possession by spirit entails the 'complete identification with the other, in the sense of having their feelings and emotions' (Skultans, 1974: 38). For the medium, there exists a loss of bodily boundaries as spirit is allowed to enter. This effectively means a temporary loss of self during which the departed are afforded an 'instrument' (the medium's body) through which to communicate: 'all the actions, both verbal and non-verbal, during possession are attributed to the possessing spirit and not to the person possessed' (ibid.: 80–81). Here the concept of control becomes crucial as it is the medium who retains command over her body and is able to force the spirit to depart. Despite the careful maintenance of the occupation of the living body, the experience of possession leads to questions regarding the identity of the medium. Spiritualist representations of the self in relation to the body are complex in that spirits of the departed are allowed to exercise their agency through a physical vessel which is successively occupied by spirits, yet ultimately controlled by the medium. As Skultans argues, 'spiritualist development implies a particular attitude to bodily control and a particular kind of relationship to the body. This involves both the renunciation of bodily control and a remote vigilance which allows for the immediate resumption of bodily control' (ibid.: 85).

During possession a medium will temporarily suffer the symptoms experienced by the spirit as an embodied being and then re-enact the, often painful, circumstances in which the person died. The medium's ritualised performance of the death scene functions to release the spirit from its earthly pain, a necessary step before the spirit is able to pass into the higher realms of the spirit world. Thus, immediately after death, spirits occupy a transitional space between the living and the dead and require the help of mediums to move beyond this dangerous phase. In Chapter 9 we made reference to the varying constructions of the boundary between life and death. For the duration of the performance, the medium is simultaneously a living and a dying body, an important site within which the dualistic life–death boundary is destabilised. This procedure which releases the distressed spirit from painful bodily sensations experienced in life is compounded when the spirit in question belongs to a deceased medium. Possession by the spirit of a former medium would imply a radical, if temporary, destabilising of the performing medium's identity. The medium therefore develops a sense of self which allows her body to be occupied by various spiritual agents. At the same time the boundaries of this self are carefully guarded in that the process of possession is controlled within ritual contexts.

Further interactions which take place at the site of the medium's body reinforce the mutual dependency of the living and the dead. During spiritualist gatherings mediums become 'impressed' by spirit. Here 'the mind is conceived of as a wax tablet upon which images or visual and auditory messages imprint themselves' (Skultans, 1974: 48). Messages are received from spirit by mediums who transmit them to the wider gathering. Skultans provides examples of message giving. Often a spirit would manifest in human form and, standing behind the person with whom it was concerned, communicate a message to the medium who would, in turn, deliver it to that person. One man was told that he had a 'gentleman of the Masonic order' behind him 'helping to shape your true self' (ibid.: 16). Other spirits were connected by kin to the recipients and some bore a physical resemblance to the living with whom they were trying to connect. In general messages were intended to provide help and advice with distress and sickness. Spiritualist encounters with the deceased are believed to provide 'mystical insight into the ordinary pains of others' (ibid.: 40). Through interaction with the spirits, physical and emotional suffering is detected and sometimes alleviated.

Communication between the living and the spirit world is predicated upon particular conceptions of the body and embodied experience. Skultans argues that 'communication at meetings has as its focus the body and onslaughts on its well-being' (1974: 35), while interest in spiritualism is expressed predominantly through the language of pain and misfortune. At the centre of spiritualist meetings there is a concern with illness and the relief of suffering. Physical ailments are interpreted as aspects of wider social and personal problems such that illness is not confined to the physical body. Rather, it is linked in crucial ways to interpersonal relationships and tensions. Each person is seen to have an 'aura', a partly physical and partly spiritual light surrounding the body, which expresses a person's social, psychological and physical well-being or 'balance' through colour. Therefore, any misfortune or problem that a person is experiencing becomes visible to the 'spiritually developed'. Therefore, the aura allows for the communication of the body's condition which is understood as an entity enmeshed in social and spiritual relations: 'physical ailments are seen to be woven into the wider fabric of other social and personal problems' (ibid.: 28). This conception of the body is crucial in spiritualist notions regarding pain and sickness. Pain is perceived as part of a private domain which is difficult to communicate and it is the use of a shared language of sickness, mobilised in spiritualist meetings, that this 'isolation' is combated. Bodily states of the living and the deceased are thereby shared. It is through possession that 'pain acquires some of the properties of a physical object, which several people can see, hear or feel at the same time' (ibid.: 37).

The focus on embodied experience is crucial to the development of mediumistic ability. Sorrow and pain, together with experiences of loss associated with the death of loved ones, increase a developing medium's sensitivity. While the majority of spiritualist gatherings are composed of women, men are valued participants and play a leading role in spirit healing. Men also occupy positions of authority in that they usually guide women in their development as mediums. During the early stages of this process a woman is considered 'inaccessible to spirit influence and unwilling to surrender her body to a spirit agency' (Skultans, 1974: 51). In this situation men will encourage women, through spirit healing, to relax and 'to let themselves go', a process which is eroticised. Gradually, mediums will learn through embodied experience to recognise and interpret the signs of spirit communication which emerge in the form of, for example, bodily heat, cold or tingling. This is a process which involves an increasing sensitivity towards physical sensation and is dependent upon the interaction and interpretation which take place within a particular social context:

> possession does not require any peculiar state of mind but rather, membership of a social group in which detailed attention is given to bodily states and in which heightened awareness of such states allows them to be identified and defined in a special way.
>
> (ibid.: 7)

Through spirit mediumship and the ritualised communication of sickness at spiritualist gatherings, the boundaries of the body and self are re-negotiated. Furthermore, agency and power reside in spirit, which is understood as 'the mystical, the non-empirical'. Such practices reproduce conceptions of embodied experience which register the interconnections between physical, social and spiritual domains. The living body, striving for health, becomes enmeshed in a network of communication which extends across the boundaries between the living and the dead. Relationships between the self and the body are reconfigured in ritual contexts through the agency of the departed. This holds for both the medium who temporarily surrenders her body to spirit agency, and other members of spiritualist gatherings who receive the attention of spirit. Skultans notes that in traditional psychiatric discourse the occupation of the body by an agent other than the self would be interpreted as a symptom of insanity. 'Loss of psychological privacy, in the sense both of sharing thoughts, emotions and feelings and having them controlled by others is taken as indicative of a loss of sanity' (1974: 39). We see a similar process at work wherever the living choose to retain such a bond with the dead. As we showed in Chapter 8, continued relationships between a widow and her dead husband are generally viewed by psychologists and bereavement counsellors as an unhealthy refusal to 'let go' and thereby reinvest in a future without the deceased.

Receptive and legible bodies

In particular performative contexts, mediums are able to provide spirits with an embodied presence which underpins and shapes the social agency of the departed. In the remainder of this chapter we discuss the ways in which contemporary clairvoyants engage with the dead through readings of the living bodies of their clients or through the use of 'tools' such as cards and crystals, again in particular ritualised contexts. We pay particular attention to the mobilisation of the body as a symbolic resource in informal rituals which operate across life/death boundaries (Hallam, 1997b). Central to this ritualised process is the receptivity of the clairvoyant's body both to images, and to the dead person, both of which are commonly regarded as 'invisible' as they belong either to the past, or to the future. Also crucial to clairvoyants' practices is the notion that the bodies of clients are legible – they are available for 'reading' and provide the basic resources which the clairvoyant uses in the selective 'telling' of the client's life story.

In the case of spiritualist groups there is a tendency towards loosely organised circles and churches which meet on a regular basis. Their beliefs and ritual practices reinforce the dynamic interaction between the living and the departed. However, in addition to these organised groups there are further informal ritual specialists who operate across life/death boundaries. In contemporary England, clairvoyants and psychics work at the local level to provide an eclectic range of services from fortune-telling to exorcism. There is a wide spectrum of practitioners who usually work on an individual basis but who also connect with spiritualist churches. For instance, Skultans observed one woman who was a regular and valued attendant at spiritualist gatherings. 'Edna' is described as a 'marginal' yet 'respected' member of a Spiritualist church who, at the age of 65, had led many services in Wales and had since developed further skills which were 'not strictly orthodox' in Spiritualist terms; namely 'second-sight', palm and crystal ball reading and psychometry. After church services Edna would use these skills in 'individual counselling services', although her practices would be considered more 'magical' than 'spiritual' (Skultans, 1974: 24). When analysing interactions between the living and the dead, therefore, we need to recognise the complexity and overlapping nature of systems of belief and practice already alluded to earlier in this chapter. There should also be acknowledgement of the diverse range of practitioners and ritual specialists who establish different modes of communication with the dead. In addition, divergent perceptions of these practitioners co-exist within any given cultural context. For instance, clairvoyants might be perceived as both tellers of significant truths and as theatrical performers. Clairvoyants themselves, sometimes play into these different roles. For example, by advertising their services in local newspapers they project themselves as skilled in private consultation, demonstration in lectures and in psychic fairs as well as party entertainment.

The gendered dimensions of clairvoyants' practices are pronounced. While Skultans notes the receptivity of men in spiritualist circles, who then teach women to open themselves out to spirit communication, we here identify women who, as clairvoyants, are perceived to be particularly sensitive and adept with regard to contact with spiritual domains. It is mostly women who become clairvoyants and, furthermore, women who make up the majority of clairvoyants' clients. We might attribute these patterns to sets of social relations and cultural assumptions which, in contemporary Western societies, reinforce gendered divisions of labour: it is usually women who become specialists dealing in the 'domestic' rituals surrounding the spheres of love, health, work and luck. One central dimension of clairvoyants' practices is their contribution to the management of life crises. They address and help to resolve clients' concerns with birth, sickness and death. There are significant comparisons to be made here with different historical and cultural contexts. For instance, in early modern England, women were directly involved in the management of rituals involved in the processes of childbirth, healing and dying (Hallam, 1994, 1996). Such ritual practices were organised and rendered meaningful within the context of women's social networks involving family, kin, neighbours and friends. The social and symbolic work undertaken by women at points of crisis and transition in the life course afforded them significant sources of authority, placing them in positions from which to challenge socially dominant gender hierarchies.

Within a different contemporary cultural setting, Serematakis explores the ritualised practices of Inner Maniat women in Greece; practices associated with death and divination. She examines these practices as 'instruments of cultural power' and 'vehicles of resistance' which provide women with a creative cultural space for the performance and articulation of their knowledge and identity (1991: 2). Tracing the related practices of death and divination from the eighteenth century, Serematakis notes that they are part of 'long-term structures which were not destroyed by modernity' (ibid.). Women have been centrally involved in mourning songs and exhumations of the dead, for example, and thus they play an important role in the management of the dead and departed body. 'These transformative practices are grounded on material forces such as pain, the body, and pollution, and creatively interact with women's experience in the economic and domestic spheres of social life' (ibid.: 2). Of particular interest here is Serematakis' account of divination which is performed by women after the exhumation of the body. The exhumed bones, and the marks they carry are interpreted in narratives and mourning songs. While the 'reading' of the bones connects them to a 'persona of the dead' (ibid.: 190), this practice also has implications for the living, as 'it is in the material evidence of the exhumed dead that the hidden acts of the living are disclosed' (ibid.: 192). Women are able to reveal socially significant, yet undisclosed, knowledge regarding relationships and activities in the community of the living. They access these truths through readings of the dead body. Serematakis points out that exhumed bones are 'not identical with the dead as agency' but that they are a 'communication device, a point of interface between the living and the dead' (ibid.: 194). Women's divinatory practices therefore mediate these domains and operate across an unstable life/death boundary. In contrast to the reading of the dead body, as described by Serematakis, stands the reading of the living body in contemporary clairvoyants' practices in England. Here we identify a process of communication which again establishes a ritualised space for interactions between the living and the dead.

The following analysis is based on the initial research results of a study which began in 1993. A large part of the ethnographic and archival research focuses on an East Midlands town where there is a common knowledge of clairvoyants who live locally and who are available to provide help with a wide range of personal anxieties and problems. It is clear from local newspapers and people's accounts that a number of clairvoyants have lived in the area from at least the mid-1950s, although comparative analysis with magical practitioners in early modern England would suggest the existence of longer-term traditions of popular belief and practice.

The wider social context in which these specialists operate is characterised by extensive networks which generate around particular clairvoyants and are often sustained for a number of years. As noted earlier, clairvoyants and their clients are mostly women. They usually hold private consultations with clients at home, although some offer to visit people and conduct readings through the post. There are also regular psychic fairs held in public houses where people can talk to clairvoyants. Faced with a wide range of local practitioners, women will make choices about who to visit based on local knowledge about particular clairvoyants' skills. Often the subject of conversation between women friends and relatives, clairvoyants acquire reputations for their accuracy and sympathetic clarity of vision. Women will often visit the same clairvoyant, returning regularly and, then recommending them to others. In this way networks of social relations are built up and sustained.

On the whole, clairvoyants are sought out by people at key stages during the life course – when relationships have broken down; when there are worries about illness, childbirth and death. In short, when the future begins to seem uncertain or when there is a degree of instability or potential change, clairvoyants are approached. Emotional upheavals, anxieties about relationships and the sickness or loss of loved ones are all referred to as issues raised during visits to clairvoyants. Phases of confusion which interrupt expectations about the continuity of events and relationships tend to threaten ontological security, destabilising a person's sense of direction. It is at these times that help may be sought from a clairvoyant. Clairvoyants sometimes refer to these phases as 'turning points' – points at which important decisions and plans are made. The invisible future, lacking in direction, appears as a potential threat, generating a perceived need for guidance and specialist advice. With their reputations for skill in these matters, clairvoyants are regularly consulted.

We might, then, identify clairvoyants as informal ritual specialists who make significant, yet socially marginalised, contributions to the management of transition and change expressed at the level of interpersonal relations and experience. Through an examination of encounters between clairvoyants and their clients, we identify clairvoyance as a cultural process which engages imaginative, emotional and embodied experience. It is also an interpretative process which hinges on the dialogic production of social meanings. In this respect clairvoyants participate in the narrative construction of self-identities and personal histories. From this theoretical perspective we here provide an account of clairvoyance in relation to concepts of the body and death.

The process of clairvoyance is expressed through a language of vision. Above all, clairvoyants render inner and intangible worlds visible. In their imaginative work they use and create images to reveal what is past and dimly perceived, what is present but somehow lacking in clarity, and what is future and therefore hidden. 'Clairvoyancy is the faculty of seeing mentally what is normally out of sight' proclaims a poster circulated by a clairvoyant in January 1994. Central to the discourse of contemporary clairvoyants is a language of the eye, of extraordinary perception within which their power of vision is represented as a way of penetrating innermost experiences, both immediate and across time. This rhetorical use of the eye – a specific bodily organ – to represent the clairvoyant's mediating capacities is not limited to a contemporary Western context. T. Lobsang Rampa, describing himself as a Tibetan monk, provides an account of how he gained access to an invisible domain – to 'see people as they are and not as they pretend to be' (Rampa: 1957: 101). This capacity came about through the surgical opening of a third eye in the flesh and bone in the middle of his forehead.

Clairvoyants will receive mental images, often of a very mundane nature, which they then communicate verbally to their client. For instance, images of people (living and deceased) and locations (houses and landscapes) associated with the client in the past as well as the present and the future.

Practices which reveal hidden knowledge can constitute significant sources of power. Tiryakian describes the process by which access to invisible domains operates through symbols. The effective manipulation of symbols to effect transformations in visible, material domains can be identified as an important aspect of clairvoyant practices. As Tiryakian argues:

> The visible world there-before-us is an ensemble of physical things, of bodies we can touch, localize, measure. The invisible world is hidden from our view. We cannot situate ourselves in relation to aspects of it in the way we can take our distance from objects in the visible world...The two worlds, however, are not in a state of radical discontinuity vis-à-vis one another. There is a 'medium' which relates the two, the medium of symbols. A 'symbol' is an empirical referent, it is capable of being grasped by the senses. It is an image, a gesture, a phrase, a physical object, etc. – anything which can act as an interchange between the two worlds, a point of contact between manifest and hidden reality. The ability to utilise these symbols, which when properly activated can harness the energy or forces of the invisible, ultimate reality to bring about changes in the conditions of the world of appearances is, at heart, a magical ability. It is an ability, obviously, not given to everyone.
>
> (1974a: 5)

The clairvoyant's powers of vision are especially significant in relation to the recovery of messages from the deceased. This is conducted in a variety of ways. For example, a clairvoyant might use 'tools' to recover images of past lives or might address spirits directly as though in conversation with them. In both situations the clairvoyant mobilises symbols, translates them into narratives and thereby attempts to provide an explanatory framework through which the client achieves a deeper understanding of their current situation. Clairvoyant/client encounters can thus be seen as a transformative process in that the client is repositioned in relation to a particular set of life problems.

Clairvoyants therefore find a role in managing life/death crises through their readings of the bodies of both the client and the spiritual 'attendants' who surround them, thereby mediating the physical and the spirit world. Clairvoyants' readings mobilise the living body as a resource through which 'spirits' are made to communicate and clients are helped with perceived life crises. The relationship between a clairvoyant and client is often mediated by a disembodied presence from the 'other' world which is visible to the clairvoyant, either directly or via a decoding of signs which emerge upon the client's body within the clairvoyant's field of vision. Such signs cluster, for example, in the lines on the palm or the face or upon objects worn about the body, such as watches. These visual clues form maps which the clairvoyant explicates, thereby constructing a narrative of the body which directs the client towards a resolution of their problems. Alternatively, a clairvoyant might read and interpret spirit messages through a range of tools including tarot cards and crystals. Here the clairvoyant will detect patterns of images emerging through this symbolic media. This reading of the body and the deciphering of signs might be compared with the ways in which women interpreted bodily signs at the death bed in different historical contexts (see Chapter 6). These processes of interpretation provide women with a measure of authority and extend their control of key transitional phases in the life course.

Death enters clairvoyant narratives in three main ways. First, a developing sensitivity to signs of the imminent death of others can be recognised as an indication that a woman is moving into her role as clairvoyant. In the reported life histories of these specialists, the ability to predict a death is acknowledged as a powerful skill which indicates to the clairvoyant that she has a distinctive capacity. Second, the clairvoyant is able to communicate with the dead. In consultations with clients the clairvoyant will detect the presence of past kin, guardians and friends, often interpreting and conveying messages from them. Such communication varies in intensity from a glimpse in a crystal to traces in the 'maps' and 'journeys' inscribed in the palm, to conversation with a 'present' spirit. Third, death appears as a metaphor in the visual culture of clairvoyancy. In the tarot deck, the death card can be read as a representation of the state of transition: death of an old state and the birth of a new one. It can refer to transformation and change in the life of the client. During a tarot reading the client has contact with the cards, often shuffling or cutting the pack. The clairvoyant will then lay out the cards in a particular pattern and from the surfacing of these images, she will compose a narrative. Dominant themes, key figures and influences which impinge on the client's current situation will be identified. This is a form of ritualised reading which connects the client to a wider context of social and personal relationships and events and in so doing offers the client a wider perspective from which to view themselves and others. Thus images relating to death and the deceased operate in significant ways in the context of clairvoyant practices.

Conclusion

Clairvoyants are seen to reveal and unveil the inner condition of their clients, their secret and emotional lives which are embedded in their past or are about to emerge. By looking at visible signs, clairvoyants are able to uncover the source of worries and problems, making them visible and meaningful to clients. They provide narratives which correspond and connect with aspects of self-identity usually conceived of as internal and private to the bounded individual. Clairvoyance is regarded as a special process of communication, during which visual images are transformed into the spoken word. Images from the body of the client, from their possessions, or from ritual objects such as cards and crystals form shapes and images which are then given meaning in relation to a particular person. Clairvoyants help to recover the past and the future within the present. Their narratives gather time together and offer the hope of control over it – in the sense that knowledge about events that have yet to unfold might enhance a person's capacity to shape them. By making the invisible future tangible, clairvoyants' stories create a route into it, a new direction that was previously unclear. These function to guide a client and in effect help to redefine the client's identity, transforming them within a therapeutic process. Central to a clairvoyant's work is the weaving of stories around visual images – these are meaningful narratives – a moment in time which makes meaning out of the conjuncture of past, present and future.

Clairvoyants' narratives draw together past, present, future and this constitutes a breakdown of temporal boundaries that situate the life/death relationship within a fixed chronology. With regard to women's ritualised practices in Inner Mani, Serematakis notes that:

> [m]astery over time in divination is at the very least an interpretative, if not instrumental, mastery over the events that occur in time and that are structured by time...To this one might add that women's temporal power is best substantiated by their control over oral history and biography.
>
> (1991, 228)

This process is further reinforced in the client's re-telling of the clairvoyant's narratives. The clairvoyant's words are sometimes tape-recorded, and women may later recount what was said to family and friends. This process of re-telling can unfold over a number of years. Women will remember what was said to them by clairvoyants in the past, invoking their words at different points in time. This is especially the case when the clairvoyant's predictions are seen to match with subsequent experience. Through ritualised readings of the body, which recover the deceased in significant ways, clairvoyants are able to access alternative sources of knowledge. The surfaces of the body, images perceived using special tools and mental images, provide a different way of perceiving the world for the clairvoyant. This field of representations, which connects embodied experience with imaginative processes, is translated into spoken accounts which are received, remembered and recounted by the client. Here we see the mediation of the living and the dead as part of a cultural practice which plays a dynamic role in the shaping of social identities and personal relationships.

Chapter 11

Beyond the body

Central to current social theories of the body is the paradox that as human beings we both have and are bodies. This work has foregrounded the fact that the bodies which we have are often taken as primary manifestations of the people we are; they are objects which play a major role in the constitution of our identities. Further, our bodies are thought of as a site within which authentic truths can be discerned, a development which, it has been suggested, reflects the diminishment of traditional sources of authority (Frank, 1990). In place of the now destabilised metanarratives of religion, nationalism or morality, we turn to the flesh for a more grounded source of knowledge. This is evidenced, for example, in the recent upsurge of interest in the influence of a genetic base in the incidence of disease, homosexuality, criminality and gendered behaviours. Going against the grain of post-war political and academic concern with the importance of the social environment, of 'nurture' rather than 'nature', this return to the body is an echo of nineteenth century theories which saw markers of criminality and madness in the face or skull shape (Lombroso, 1911).

This belief that the body can provide foundational knowledge has been identified by theorists working from a Foucauldian or discursive position. Alongside this prioritising of body-based knowledge they have also highlighted the historical mutability of knowledges of the body. As metanarratives, such belief systems may be professional, academic or lay: a formal classification of blood types or skull sizes; a theory of evolution based on recovered skeletal material; a framework of ideas about the causes of colds or the cut of clothing. They may be formulated as an explicit system or realised only as a form of practical mastery which lies beyond cognition or verbal articulation (Bourdieu, 1977). According to this view, therefore, aspects of the body which we take as essential to its 'nature', reflect particular ideologies which are brought into play through discourses and social practices. In other words, the body-as-knowledge-source is but one among many constructions or readings of the flesh. This view remains powerful as a perspective from which to think critically about the ways in which the members of certain social categories come to be positioned, socially, politically and economically, on the basis of sets of assumptions which reside largely within or on the body. The capacity of a discursive approach to destabilise those knowledges which are felt to be lodged within the flesh has made it attractive to sociologists with interests as varied as consumption, disability, feminist theory, medicine, health and illness and criminality. Its critics argue, however, that it is limited as a way of understanding the bodies which we are. That is, it allows us to think about the objectification of the body but fails in phenomenological terms to provide a full and sufficient account of being and having a body. Being discursively produced, the bodies which we 'think' we have are in danger of 'de-materialising' as we come to realise, for example, that the diseases which our GPs diagnose are but the product of a particular classificatory system.

This volume has focused on the body in crisis, in illness and deterioration, death and disposal. Discursive theories have been important to the perspectives we have developed here; for example, in allowing us to describe the progressive objectification of the body. As we have shown, in younger, healthy adulthood, the body disappears from consciousness. In childhood, by contrast, we may experience our bodies with some intensity in that they are too small for the adult world of furniture, staircases, public transport and toilets. Either we stand on tip-toes or we manage with modifications – car seats, toilet seats, buggies, prams and play pens. The bodily skills needed to manipulate a cultural and social environment designed for adults are similarly elusive for children; for example, despite their unparalleled ability to suck the nipple, they are made dependent upon the complex paraphernalia of lidded cups, heated plates, high chairs, reinforced bibs and crooked spoons in order to participate in contemporary, adult eating practices. As adults, however, our bodies can disappear into an environment which smoothly accommodates their needs. The skills with which we can manage our body, deploying it as a resource which reveals our good taste, our athletic prowess, our personal magnetism, are 'privately' learned, their aim being to present our bodies as intrinsically, indeed effortlessly, healthy, well groomed and slim. Surgically produced beauty, for example, remains troubling for many Westerners. Orlan, the performance artist, has made an impact by disrupting the silence within which adults manage their individual bodies-as-objects. By televising a sequence of elective surgical operations upon her body, she confronts her audiences with her own flesh as the object which she chooses to act upon as a medium for artistic expression. Hers is an artistic endeavour which profoundly troubles the viewer, not only at the visceral level of witnessing another individual opt for pain, but also at a conceptual level. Her televised performances demonstrate unequivocally that the body is an object, one which she chooses to act upon directly (Davis, 1997).

Managed in culturally prescribed silence and privacy, however, our adult bodies are objects through which we enhance our status in the eyes of family, friends and colleagues. It is in illness or later life that they again become objects from which we may feel alienated. They stand apart from our sense of our selves, constituting ungovernable misrepresentations of the people we know ourselves to be. Increasingly visible, both to us and to those around us, our bodies can make us susceptible to forms of surveillance, either from younger family members who fear that our standards of housework, personal hygiene or ability to safely negotiate the external environment may be inadequate, or from employers, health visitors, social workers and doctors who share these same concerns. It is in death that the object-like nature of the body becomes most visible. Rather than the smoothly managed object which, as adults with social and economic resources at our disposal, we can dress and position in socially advantageous ways, our dead body lies totally beyond our control, shamefully breaching the boundaries over which, since earliest childhood, we learn to maintain vigilant control. As Chapter 7 has shown, the dead body attracts stigma and inspires fear, its inevitable deterioration revealing it as the object we once had rather the individual we once were. Via the services of the undertaker the body again, briefly, is made to reflect the person we have been. It is this representation, constructed at the site of the body which, like the performance art of Orlan, uses the flesh as a creative medium. Importantly, as argued in Chapter 7, it is one which conceals rather than reveals the mechanisms through which it has been produced. In the case of Orlan we see the flesh of a conscious woman being cut open. Hence its power to shock us by dramatising the normally hidden practices through which we manage the object/bodies which we have. Muffling the shock of a death, however, undertakers are at pains to disguise the violence which they inflict upon the flesh in their efforts to re-construct the person it once was. When safely re-presented at the site of the corpse, relatives and friends come to witness a 'memory picture' which can then sustain the future social life of the now disembodied individual.

Discursive theories therefore take us a long way in helping to make sense of the progressively problematic objectification of the body. The concept of 'social death', which we have drawn upon repeatedly throughout this book, is an example of a perspective which highlights the deleterious effects of externally imposed ideologies and assumptions. Yet, as discussed in Chapter 3, the objectification of the body, implied by models such as the mask of ageing (Featherstone and Hepworth, 1991), highlights a splitting between body and self which, though illuminating, can be a difficult theoretical position from which to explore the subjective experience of being a body. If we wish to better account for the materiality of the discursively constructed body, we can turn to Csordas' notion of 'being-in-the-world' as a way of addressing the immediacy of sensual embodied experience. The recent emphasis on embodiment as a way of reconciling discursive and materialist accounts of the body has been effective to an extent. Shilling's identification of the 'finishing' of the body pinpoints the social processes through which the flesh is humanised (1993). Turner uses the terms 'enselvement' to similarly describe the processes through which the flesh is gradually experienced as, and made to represent the self (1998).

The materials we have been examining in some detail through-out this book cannot, however, be adequately theorised using any of the terms set out above. They will not do the job with sufficient precision. Our agenda in writing this book therefore reflects a tradition of developing theory by moving back and forth between abstract schema and localised data (Geertz, 1977). Working with our own empirical and archival findings, and those of other social scientists in the field of death, dying and bereavement, we became aware of limitations within current social theories of the body and were stimulated to begin re-casting ideas about body and self along different lines. Just as encounters with mortality have traditionally precipitated a re-visioning of the values and priorities seen as central to 'life' (see Chapter 2), so work on the body in crisis challenges many of the assumptions which underpin theories of the body in everyday life.

In this final chapter of the book, we draw together those data which challenge these assumptions. Chapter 1 argued that at the margins of social life, the elision of self and body – or, discursively, multiple selves and multiple bodies – becomes highly complex. Bodies can be made to survive accidents or the conditions of extreme age, almost in the absence of the self, so constituting a hybrid category of inanimate but living object – the 'vegetable'. And, paradoxically, our data show that the self, which we increasingly conceive of as an embodied entity, can retain social presence and indeed agency after the death and disposal of the flesh. This may occur via the sense of an intimate domestic presence, the manifesta-tion of a ghost or the evocation of a spirit at the site of a client or clairvoyant's body. Powerfully felt, yet conceptually beyond the limits of Western empiricism, the dead have a hybrid existence. Their categorical ambiguity is epitomised in the horror narrative of the living/dead vampire which preys upon the living, drawing out their 'life' in the form of blood yet re-animating their 'dead' bodies. Examining the more mundane setting of a residential home for older adults, the relationship between the old body and the self remains elusive. As Chapter 3 showed, this material highlights a lack of consensus within current social theories of the body. Does later life embodiment represent a final, intense period of 'enselvement'? Or can it better be understood as an experience of bodily objectification, the younger self remaining alive in memory behind the 'mask' of ageing? Or can a form of psychic death occur which empties the object/body of the self? Discursive perspectives might illuminate the openness of the old body to a multiplicity of readings; but they shed less light on the subjective experience of embodiment in later life. Crucially, these theoretical approaches rest upon the assumption that body and self are one and the same thing and that conditions such as extreme old age, brain damage or brain death bring about aberrant conjugations of self and body. If the injured or very elderly individual's family continue to incorporate them within everyday social life, they are thought to be spuriously retaining the illusion of a surviving self – either at the site of the PVS body or via re-embodiment in the form of donated organs. However, if they take as 'dead' the older adult who is beyond the social interaction of earlier years, if they grieve the loss of the individual they once loved, this raises the spectre of human beings ageing and dying as 'objectified' entities which can only be 'warehoused' (Miller and Gwynne, 1972). Younger adults must therefore live not only with the prospect of their own mortality, but also the risk of becoming a corpse which the undertaker cruelly omits to collect (Miller, 1990).

In positing the body as discursively constructed rather than biologically given, theorists working from a Foucauldian perspective also highlight the possibility of a multiplicity of bodies, subsumed within what appears to be one flesh. This was evidenced among the stillborn babies discussed in Chapter 4. Their status as dead matter, the unwanted products of conception or a dead son or daughter was variously interpreted by professionals and parents. Differences not only separated one professional from another, but also emerged within interview data from a parent who might feel both fear of a corpse as well as love for a son or daughter. Ambiguities were also evidenced in relation to the status of transplanted organs and the bodies of brain-dead patients, in that it was not clear whether they were dead matter or viable social beings. This approach takes us some way towards making sense of experiences of, and associated with, the body in crisis. If we work from a post-structuralist model of a decentred or fragmented self, then the notion of a body which is amenable to multiple, synchronic readings is an unproblematic part of the same theoretical picture. However, the data we are working with raise even more fundamental questions about the assumptions which underpin current theories of the body.

This book moves 'beyond the body' not just in a substantive sense – that is, not simply by extending its focus into the period which comes after bodily demise. Certainly the scope of its material is far broader than that encompassed within many death studies' publications where there is a tendency either to examine terminal illness, or death ritual or grief mechanisms. It is a diversity of focus which often reflects a disciplinary fragmentation between palliative medicine, social anthropology, sociology and psychiatry. We suggest that this inclination towards substantive and discipline-based specialisation among scholars of death and dying has costs. We also suggest that there are costs to a social theory of the body which rarely ventures beyond the limits of adulthood. This book therefore makes a strong theoretical claim that any account of what it means to be human must not only attend to the embodied nature of this experience, but also crucially move beyond the body to take account of shared, inter-subjective embodiment: for example, between a clairvoyant, her client and a relative who has 'gone before', between an organ recipient and an accident victim, between an older widow and her deceased partner. And if we problematise models of an individuated self, we also begin to destabilise the model of enselvement which would fasten the individual into a single container body and make this a primary source of self-identity. As the later chapters in this volume have demonstrated, self-identity frequently extends beyond the body. These data represent a profound challenge to a sociology which privileges face-to-face social interaction and limits itself to a model of society made up, for example, of 'workers', 'families', 'professionals', 'governments', and so on. Social anthropologists may have taken more interest in society's dead members, but significantly, these dead rarely challenge Western eschatologies, being the safely distanced members of more traditional societies. It might seem that the dead members of contemporary Western society have little scope for any post-mortem influence upon, or place within the world. The families who might remember them may well become increasingly fragmented; the value of their achievements is unlikely to be sustained, given the speed of social change. It is this view which, arguably, informs the work of theorists who highlight the ultimately futile nature of human social life and point towards culture as a desperate bulwark erected in the face of otherwise terrifying meaninglessness and oblivion (Bauman, 1992; Seale, 1998).

However, if we look more directly at the body in crisis via the data presented here, we begin to feel confined or even claustrophobic when faced with this kind of argument. In repairing the omission of the body from social theory, sociologists have been tempted into an alliance with dominant representations of the body, many of which constitute a commoditisation of bodies as temporarily desirable objects for consumption. Once the relationship between body and self-identity becomes radically destabilised, as in the data presented here, we can begin to engage with a deeper sociality which goes beyond the body. And in so doing, the privileging of biological death as an end point beyond which society's members may not stray, becomes questionable. Indeed, as these data indicate, the relationship between the concept of 'death' and the particular bodily changes which we call 'dying', is highly mutable. It is the confinement of our gaze to the body alone which produces forms of binaristic thinking within which 'life' and 'death', as biologically based categories, come to stand in a clear and oppositional relationship to one another. Once we move beyond the body we are freed up to take a more far reaching and encompassing view of human sociality. The material which forms the core of this book represents a relatively marginalised area within dominant academic or medical discourses; mainstream social scientists have, for example, had little to say about embalming, exorcism or clairvoyance. Moreover, these spheres of interest constitute sub-headings within the domain of death and dying, a field itself commonly trivialised, neglected or exoticised (Kelleher, 1995). We argue that the voices, practices and experiences encompassed within these data demand our attention. They testify to a complexity of experience around death, dying and the body in crisis which cannot be reduced simply to a body-based dualism.

Bibliography

Agich, G.J. (1983) 'Disease and value: a rejection of the value-neutrality thesis', *Theoretical Medicine*, 4, 27–41.

Arber, S. and Ginn, J. (1991) *Gender and Later Life*, London: Sage.

Ariès, P. ([1977] 1983) *The Hour of Our Death*, London: Penguin.

Armitage, S. (1998) *All Points North*, London: Viking.

Armstrong, A. (1987) 'Foucault and the problem of human anatomy', in G. Scambler (ed.) *Sociological Theory and Medical Sociology*, London: Tavistock.

Armstrong, D. (1981) 'Pathological life and death: medical spatialisation and geriatrics', *Social Science and Medicine*, 15 (A), 253–258.

——(1983) *The Political Anatomy of the Body*, Cambridge: Cambridge University Press.

Arnason, A. (1998) ' "Feel the Pain": death, grief and bereavement counselling in the North East of England', unpublished PhD thesis, University of Durham.

Arnold, K. and McKee, F. (1997) 'Doctor Death: the exhibition', in K. Arnold, B. Hurwitz, F. McKee and R. Richardson (eds) *Doctor Death. Medicine at the End of Life*, London: The Wellcome Trust.

Asad, T. (1998) 'Agency, subject, the body', plenary address, After the Body Conference, University of Manchester.

Badham, P. (1989) 'Does religion need immortality?', in A. Berger, P. Badham, A.H. Kutscher, J. Berger, M. Perry and J. Beloff (eds) *Perspectives on Death and Dying; Cross-Cultural and Multi-Disciplinary Views*, Philadelphia: the Charles Press.

Bakhtin, M.M. (1981) *The Dialogic Imagination. Four Essays by M. M. Bakhtin*, edited by M. Holquist, translated by C. Emerson and M. Holquist, Austin, TX: University of Texas Press.

Ball, M. (1976) *Death*, London: Oxford University Press.

Barthes, R. (1973) *Mythologies*, London: Granada.

Bartlett, E.T. (1995) 'Differences between death and dying', *Journal of Medical Ethics*, 21, 270–276.

Battersby, C. (1993) 'Her body/her boundaries. Gender and the metaphysics of containment', *Journal of Philosophy and the Visual Arts*, pp 31–39.

Bauby, J-D. (1997) *The Diving-Bell and the Butterfly*, London: Fourth Estate.

Bauman, Z. (1992) *Mortality, Immortality and Other Life Strategies*, Cambridge: Polity Press.

Beaver, D. (1992) ' "Sown in dishonour, raised in glory": death, ritual and social organization in Northern Gloucestershire, 1590–1690', *Social History*, 17, 399–419.

Becker, A. (1995) *Body, Self and Society. A View from Fiji*, Philadelphia: University of Pennsylvania Press.

Becker, H. (1963) *Outsiders: studies in the sociology of deviance*, Glencoe, Illinois: Free Press

Beer, G. (1996) ' "Authentic tidings of invisible things": vision and the invisible in the later nineteenth century', in T. Brennan and M. Jay (eds) *Vision in Context. Historical and Contemporary Perspectives on Sight*, London: Routledge.

Beier, L. M. (1989) 'The good death in seventeenth-century Great Britain', in R. Houlbrooke (ed.) *Death, Ritual and Bereavement*, London: Routledge.

Bennett, G. (1985) 'Heavenly protection and family unity: the concept of the revenant among elderly urban women', *Folklore*, 96, 87–97.

Binski, P. (1996): *Medieval Death. Ritual and Representation*, London: British Museum Press.

Bloch, M. ([1971] 1994) *Placing the Dead. Tombs, Ancestral Villages, and Kinship Organization in Madgascar*, Illinois, Waveland Press Inc.

——(1982) 'Death, women and power', in M. Bloch and J. Parry (eds), *Death and the Regeneration of Life*, Cambridge: Cambridge University Press.

Bloch, M. and Parry, J. (1982) *Death and the Regeneration of Life*, Cambridge: Cambridge University Press.

Borin, F. (1993) 'Judging by images', in N.Z. Davis and A. Farge (eds) *A History of Women III. Renaissance and Enlightenment Paradoxes*, Cambridge, MA: The Belknap Press of Harvard University Press, pp. 187–254.

Boughton, M. (1997) 'Embodied self, human biology and experience', in J. Lawler (ed.) *The Body in Nursing*, Melbourne: Churchill Livingstone.

Bourdieu, P. (1977) *Outline of a Theory of Practice*, Cambridge: Cambridge University Press.

Bourke, J. (1996) *Dismembering the Male. Men's Bodies, Britain and the Great War*, London: Reaktion Books Ltd.

Bowker, J. (1991) *The Meanings of Death*, Cambridge: Cambridge University Press.

Bowlby, J. (1980) *Attachment and Loss*, Vol. 3, New York: Basic Books.

Brodrick Committee (1971) *Report of the Committee on Death Certification and Coroners*, Cmnd. 4810, London: HMSO.

Bronfen, E. (1992) *Over Her Dead Body. Death, Femininity and the Aesthetic*, Manchester: Manchester University Press.

Bronfen, E. and Goodwin, S. W. (1993) 'Introduction', in Bronfen, E. and Goodwin, S.W. *Death and Representation*, Baltimore: The Johns Hopkins Press, pp. 3–25.

Bruce, S. (1996) *Religion in the Modern World. From Cathedrals to Cults*, Oxford: Oxford University Press.

Butler, J. (1993) *Bodies that Matter: On the Discursive Limits of 'Sex'*, London: Routledge.

Camille, M. (1994) 'The image and the self: unwriting late medieval bodies', in S. Kay and M. Rubin (eds) *Framing Medieval Bodies*, Manchester: Manchester University Press, 62–99.

(CCAL) Canterbury Cathedral Archives and Library, *Canterbury Church Court Depositions*, references as shown.

Carey, T. (1639) *The Mirror Which Flatters Not*, London: R. Thale, reprinted in E. and J. Lehner (1971) *Devils, Demons and Damnation*, New York: Dover Publications Inc.

Cohen, A. and Rapport, N. (1995) *Questions of Consciousness*, London: Routledge.

Conway, S. and Hockey, J. (1998) 'Resisting the " mask" iof old age?: the social meaning of lay health beliefs in later life', *Ageing and Society*, 18, 469–494.

Coward, R. (1984) *Female Desire*, London: Paladin.

Creed, B. (1995) 'Horror and the carnivalesque: the body-monstrous', in L. Devereaux and R. Hillman (eds) *Fields of Vision: Essays in Film Studies, Visual Anthropology and Photography*, Berkeley, CA: University of California Press, 127–159.

Cressy, D. (1989) 'Death and the social order: the funerary preferences of Elizabethan gentlemen', in *Continuity and Change* 5, 99–120.

——(1997) *Birth, Marriage and Death. Ritual, Religion and the Life-Cycle in Tudor and Stuart England*, Oxford: Oxford University Press.

Crombie, A. (1997) 'Organ and tissue donation: issues and choices', Paper presented at the Nursing Times National Conference, Death: A Living Issue, Kensington Town Hall, London.

Csordas, T. (1994) *Embodiment and Experience*, Cambridge: Cambridge University Press.

——(1996) 'A handmaid's tale: the rhetoric of personhood in American and Japanese healing of abortions', in C.F. Sargent and C.B. Brettell (eds) *Gender and Health*, Englewood Cliffs, NJ: Prentice-Hall.

Davis, K. (1995) *Reshaping the Female Body. The Dilemma of Cosmetic Surgery*, New York, Routledge.

——(1997) ' "My body is my art": cosmetic surgery as feminist utopia', in K. Davis (ed.) *Embodied Practices: Feminist Perspectives on the Body*, London, Sage.

Douglas, M. (1966) *Purity and Danger: An Analysis of the Concepts of Pollution and Taboo*, London: Routledge and Kegan Paul.

Du Boulay, J. (1982) 'The Greek vampire: a study of cyclic symbolism in marriage and death', *Man*, XVII, 219–238.

Evans-Pritchard, E. (1937) *Witchcraft, Oracles and Magic among the Azande*, Oxford: Oxford University Press.

Featherstone, M. (1995) 'The body in consumer culture', in M. Featherstone, M. Hepworth and B.S. Turner (eds) *The Body: Social Process and Cultural Theory*, London: Sage.

Featherstone, M. and Hepworth, M. (1991) 'The mask of ageing and the postmodern life course', in M. Featherstone, M. Hepworth and B.S. Turner (eds) *The Body: Social Process and Cultural Theory*, London: Sage.

Featherstone, M. and Wernick, A. (eds) *Images of Aging: Cultural Representations of Later Life*, London: Routledge.

Field, D. (1996) 'Awareness and modern dying', *Mortality*, 1(3), 255–267.

Finucane, R.C. (1996) *Ghosts: Appearances of the Dead and Cultural Transformation*, New York: Prometheus Books.

Fischler, C. (1974) 'Astrology and French society: the dialectic of archaism and modernity', in E.A. Tiryakian (ed.) *On the Margins of the Visible. Sociology, the Esoteric, and the Occult*, New York: John Wiley & Sons.

Fletcher, A. (1995) *Gender, Sex and Subordination in England, 1500–1800*, New Haven: Yale University Press.

Foucault, M. (1973) *The Birth of the Clinic: An Archaeology of Medical Perception*, London: Tavistock.

——(1977) *Discipline and Punish: Birth of the Prison*, London: Tavistock.

Frank, A. (1990) 'Bringing bodies back in: a decade review', *Theory, Culture and Society*, 7, 131–162.

Geary, P. (1986) 'Sacred commodities: the circulation of medieval relics', in A. Appadurai (ed.) *The Social Life of Things. Commodities in Cultural Perspective*, Cambridge: Cambridge University Press.

Geertz, C. (1977) 'From the native's point of view', in J.L. Dolgin, D.S. Kemnilzer and D.M. Schneider (eds) *Symbolic Anthropology*, New York: Columbia University Press.

Giddens, A. (1991) *Modernity and Self Identity*, Cambridge: Polity Press.

Gillis, J. (1997) *A World of the Own Making*, Oxford: Oxford University Press.

Gittings, C. (1984) *Death, Burial and the Individual in Early Modern England*, London: Croom Helm.

Glaser, B. and Strauss, A. (1965) *Awareness of Dying*, Chicago: Aldine.

——(1968) *Time for Dying*, Chicago: Aldine.

Glob, P.V. (1977) *The Bog People: Iron-Age Man Preserved*, Chatham: Faber and Faber.

Goffman, E. (1959) *The Presentation of Self in Everyday Life*, New York: Doubleday.

Gorer, G. (1965) *Death, Grief and Mourning in Contemporary Britain*, London: Cresset.

Grosz, E. (1989) *Sexual Subversions*, St Leonards, Australia: Allen and Unwin.

Grosz, E. and Probyn, E. (eds) (1995) *Sexy Bodies: The Strange Carnalities of Feminism*, London: Routledge.

Hallam, E. (1994) 'Crisis and representation: gender and social relations in Canterbury and its region, 1580–1640', unpublished PhD thesis, University of Kent at Canterbury.

——(1996) 'Turning the hourglass: gender relations at the deathbed in early modern Canterbury', *Mortality*, 1(1), 61–82.

——(1997a) 'Death and the transformation of gender in image and text', in D. Field, J. Hockey and N. Small (eds.) *Death, Gender and Ethnicity*, London: Routledge, 108–123.

——(1997b) 'Clairvoyants, death and visual culture in England', The Social Context of Death, Dying and Disposal, Third International Conference, University of Wales, Cardiff, unpublished paper.

Hammerton, J.A. (undated) 'War graves', in J.A. Hammerton (ed.), *Harmsworth's Universal Encyclopedia*, Vol. 9, London: The Amalgamated Press Ltd.

Harrison, T. (1993) *Black Daisies for the Bride*, London: Faber.

Heald, M. with Brown, S. (1994) *Care for Bereaved Parents: An Evaluative Study: A Research Action Report*, commissioned by CFBP Management Committee, Middlesborough: Inhouse Publication.

Helman, C. (1990) *Culture, Health and Illness*, Oxford: Butterworth: Heinemann.

Hertz, R. ([1907] 1960) *Death and the Right Hand*, New York: Free Press.

Hinton, J. (1967) *Dying*, reprinted 1984, Harmondsworth: Penguin.

Hockey, J. (1990) *Experiences of Death: An Anthropological Account*, Edinburgh: Edinburgh University Press.

——(1992) *Making the Most of a Funeral*, London: Cruse-Bereavement Care.

——(1996) 'Encountering the "reality of death" through professional discourses: the matter of materiality', *Mortality*, 1 (1), 45–60.

——(1999) 'Houses of doom', in T. Chapman and J. Hockey (eds) *Ideal Homes*, London: Routledge.

Hockey, J. and James, A. (1993) *Growing Up and Growing Old: Ageing and Dependency across the Lifecourse*, London, Sage.

Houlbrooke, R.A. (1979) *Church Courts and the People during the English Reformation, 1520–1570*, Oxford: Oxford University Press.

——(ed.) (1989) *Death, Ritual and Bereavement*, London: Routledge.

Howarth, G. (1994) 'Quality of life study', unpublished research data, funded by the Nuffield Foundation.

——(1995) 'Elderly women caring for a dying spouse', unpublished paper, Gender and Ageing Conference, University of Surrey.

——(1996) *Last Rites: The Work of the Modern Funeral Director*, New York: Baywood Publishing Company.

——(1997) 'Death on the road: the role of the English coroner's court in the social construction of an accident', in M. Mitchell (ed.) *The Aftermath of Road Accidents: Psychological, Social and Legal Consequences of an Everyday Trauma*, London: Routledge.

——(1998) ' "Just live for today": living, caring, ageing and dying', *Ageing and Society*, 18, 6, 673–89.

Huizinga, J. (1954) *The Waning of the Middle Ages*, New York: Doubleday.

Huntington, R. and Metcalf, P. (1979) *Celebrations of Death. The Anthropology of Mortuary Ritual*, Cambridge: Cambridge University Press.

Illich, I. (1976) *Medical Nemesis: The Expropriation of Health*, London: Marion Boyars.

Jay, M. (1996) 'Vision in context: reflections and refractions', in T. Brennan and M. Jay (eds) *Vision in Context; Historical and Contemporary Perspectives on Sight*, London: Routledge, 1–14.

Jenks, C. (ed.) (1995) *Visual Culture*, London: Routledge.

——(1998) *Core Sociological Dichotomies*, London: Sage.

Jones, A. R. (1987) 'Nets and bridles: early modern conduct books and sixteenth-century women's lyrics', in N. Armstrong and L. Tennenhouse (eds) *The Ideology of Conduct: Essays in Literature and the History of Sexuality*, London: Methuen, 39–72

Jorgensen, D.L. and Jorgensen, L. (1982) 'Social meanings of the occult', *The Sociological Quarterly*, Summer, 373–389.

Jupp, P.C. (1990) *From Dust to Ashes: The Replacement of Burial by Cremation in England, 1840–1967*, London: The Congregational Lecture.

——(1993) 'The development of cremation in England, 1820–1990: a sociological account', unpublished PhD thesis, University of London.

Kellaher, L., Francis, D. and Neophytou, G. (1998) 'A bridge between two worlds', unpublished conference paper, The Social Context of Death, Dying and Disposal, 4th International Conference, Glasgow.

Kellehear, A. (1995) 'Sociology and the near-death experience', plenary address, 2nd International Conference on the Social Context of Death, Dying and Disposal, University of Sussex.

——(1996) *Experiences Near Death*, New York and Oxford: Oxford University Press.

Keller, M. (1998) 'How postcolonial bodies have redefined religious studies', Paper given at the After the Body Conference, University of Manchester.

Klass, D. (1984) 'Bereaved parents and The Compassionate Friends: affiliation and healing', *Omega, Journal of Death and Dying Studies*, 15 (4), 353–373.

Klass, D., Silverman, P. and Nickman, S. (1996) *Continuing Bonds. New Understandings of Grief*, Washington: Taylor & Francis.

Kleinman, A. (1988) *The Illness Narratives: Suffering, Healing and the Human Condition*, New York: Basic Books.

Komaromy, C. and Hockey, J. (in press) ' "Natural" death among older adults in residential care', in J. Hockey, J. Katz and N. Small (eds) *Grief, Mourning and Death Ritual*, Buckingham: Open University Press.

Kristeva, J. (1982) *Powers of Horror. An Essay on Abjection*, New York: Columbia University Press.

Lambek, M. (1996) 'Afterword: spirits and their histories', in J.M. Mageo and A. Howard (eds) *Spirits in Culture, History and Mind*, London: Routledge.

Laws, S. (1990) *Issues of Blood: The Politics of Menstruation*, Basingstoke: Macmillan.

Lawton, J. (1998) 'Contemporary hospice care: the sequestration of the unbounded body and "dirty dying" ', *Sociology of Health and Illness*, 20 (2): 121–143.

Lehner, E.J. (1971) *Devils, Demons, Death and Damnation*, New York: Dover Publications.

Lévi-Strauss, C. (1973) *Tristes Tropiques*, London: Jonathan Cape.

Levy, R.I. *et al.* (1996) 'Gods, spirits and history: a theoretical perspective', in J.M. Mageo and A. Howard (eds) *Spirits in Culture, History and Mind*, London: Routledge.

Lincoln, B. 1989) *Discourse and the construction of society : comparative studies of myth, ritual, and classification*, Oxford: Oxford University Press.

Llewellyn, N. (1991) *The Art of Death: Visual Culture in the English Death Ritual, 1500–1800*, London: Reaktion Books.

Lombroso, C. (1911) *Crime: Its Causes and Remedies*, Boston: Little Brown.

Long, M. (1984) 'Testament to a dead daughter', *The Sunday Times*, 18 November.

Lovell, A. (1983) 'Some questions of identity: late miscarriage, stillbirth and perinatal death, *Social Science and Medicine*, 17 (7), 55–61.

——(1997) 'Death at the beginning of life', in D. Field, J. Hockey and N. Small (eds) *Death, Gender and Ethnicity*, London: Routledge.

Luhrmann, T.M. (1989) *Persuasions of the Witch's Craft. Ritual Magic in Contemporary England*, Cambridge, MA: Harvard University Press.

Lupton, D. (1996) 'The imperative of health', in A. Peterson and D. Lupton (eds) *The New Public Health: Health and Self in the Age of Risk*, St Leonards, NSW: Allen & Unwin.

McCann, G. (1991) 'Biographical boundaries: sociology and Marilyn Monroe', in M. Featherstone *et al.* (eds) *The Body. Social Process and Cultural Theory*, London: Sage.

Marwit, S.J. and Klass, D. (1994) 'Grief and the role of the inner representation of the deceased', *Omega, Journal of Death and Dying Studies*, 30 (4), 283–289.

Matthews, P. and Foreman, J. (1993) *Jervis on the Office and Duties of Coroners*, 11th edn, London: Sweet & Maxwell.

Matthews, S. (1979) *The Social World of Old Women: Management of self Identity*, Beverly Hills: Sage.

Matus, J.L. (1995) *Unstable Bodies. Victorian Representations of Sexuality and Maternity,* Manchester: Manchester University Press.

Mauss, M. (1973 [1934]) 'Techniques of the body', *Economy and Society*, 2, 70–88.

Mellor, P.A. and Shilling, C. (1997) *Re-forming the Body: Religion, Community and Modernity*, London: Sage.

Merleau-Ponty, M. (1962) *Phenomology of Perception*, London: Routledge and Kegan Paul.

Miller, E.J. and Gwynne, G.V. (1972) *A Life Apart: A Pilot Study of Residential Institutions for the Physically Handicapped and Young Chronically Sick*, London: Tavistock.

Miller, J. (1990) Interview in R. Dinnage (ed.) *The Ruffian on the Stairs*, Harmondsworth: Penguin.

Mitford, J. (1963) *The American Way of Death*, London: Hutchinson.

Moss, M.S. and Moss, S.Z. (1996) 'Remarriage of widowed persons: a triadic relationship', in D. Klass *et al.* (eds) *Continuing Bonds: New Understandings of Grief*, Washington, DC: Taylor & Francis.

Moore, H. (1994) *A Passion for Difference*, Cambridge: Polity Press.

Mulkay, M. (1993) 'Social death in Britain', Sociological Review Monograph, No. 40, (ed.) D. Clark *The Sociology of Death*, 31–50.

Mulkay, M. and Ernst, J. (1991) 'The changing profile of social death', *European Journal of Sociology*, 32, 172–196.

Myerhoff, B. G. (1978) *Number Our Days*, New York: Dutton.

National Association of Funeral Directors (1988) *Manual of Funeral Directing*, London: NAFD.

Nettleton, S. (1996) 'Women and the new paradigm of health and medicine', *Critical Social Policy*, 48.

——(1998) *The Body in Everyday Life*, London: Routledge.

Okely, J. (1983) *The Traveller Gypsies*, Cambridge: Cambridge University Press.

——(1996) 'Fortune-tellers, fakes or therapists', in *Own or Other Culture*, London: Routledge.

Oppenheim, J. (1985) *The Other World. Spiritualism and Psychical research in England, 1850–1914*, Cambridge, Cambridge University Press.

Parkes, C.M. (1986) *Bereavement: Studies of Grief in Adult Life*, London: Tavistock.

Parkin, D. (1992) 'Ritual as spatial direction and bodily division', in D. De Coppet (ed.) *Understanding Rituals*, London: Routledge.

Parsons, T. (1951) *The Social System*, New York: Free Press.

Pascall, G. (1997) *Social Policy: A New Feminist Analysis*, London: Routledge.

Picardie, J. (1997) 'Before she said goodbye', *Observer Life*, 28 September.

Pine, V.R. (1975) *Caretaker of the Dead: The American Funeral Director*, New York: Irvington.

Porter, R. (1991) 'History of the body', in P. Burke (ed.) *New Perspectives on Historical Writing*, Cambridge: Polity Press.

Prior, L. (1989) *The Social Organization of Death: Medical Discourse and Social Practices in Belfast*, Basingstoke: Macmillan.

Prout, A. (ed.) (forthcoming) *The Body, Childhood and Society*, Basingstoke: Macmillan.

Radley, A. (1994) *Making Sense of Illness*, London: Sage.

Rampa, T.L. (1957) *The Third Eye: The Autobiography of a Tibetan Lama*, London: Secker & Warburg.

Rando, T. (1992) 'The increasing prevalence of complicated mourning: the onslaught is just beginning', *Omega, Journal of Death and Dying Studies*, 26 (1), 43–59.

Rees, W.D. (1971) 'The hallucinations of widowhood', *British Medical Journal*, 4, 4.

Revel, (1989) 'The uses of civility', in R. Chartier (ed.) *A History of Private Life III. Passions of the Renaissance*, Cambridge, MA: The Belknap Press of Harvard University Press.

Richardson, R. (1987) *Death, Dissection and the Destitute*, London: Routledge and Kegan Paul.

Riches, G. and Dawson, P. (1997) ' "Shoring up the walls of heartache": parental responses to the death of a child', in D. Field, J. Hockey and N. Small (eds) *Death, Gender and Ethnicity*, London: Routledge.

Roberts, R. (1997) 'Taxonomy: some notes towards the histories of photography and classification', in C. Iles and R. Roberts (eds) *In Visible Light. Photography and Classification in Art, Science and the Everyday*, Oxford: Museum of Modern Art, Oxford, 9–53.

Robbins, M. (1996) 'The donation of organs for transplantation: the donor families', in G. Howarth and P.C. Jupp (eds) *Contemporary Issues in the Sociology of Death, Dying and Disposal*, Basingstoke: Macmillan.

Rock, P. (1997) *After Homicide*, Oxford: Clarendon Press.

Rosaldo, R. (1989) *Culture and Truth: The Remaking of Social Analysis*, Boston: Beacon Press.

Ruby, J. (1995): *Secure the Shadow: Death and Photography in America*, Cambridge, MA: The MIT Press.

Sawday, J. (1995) *The Body Emblazoned. Dissection and the Human Body in Renaissance Culture*, London: Routledge.

Schafer, R. (1989) 'Dead faces', in *Granta* 27, Death, Summer 1989, Middlesex: Granta Publications Ltd, 193–210.

Seale, C. (1998) 'The body and death', Making Sense of the Body, BSA Conference, Edinburgh, unpublished paper.

Serematakis, C.N. (1991) *The Last Word: Women, Death and Divination in Inner Mani*, Chicago: Chicago University Press.

Shilling, C. (1993) *The Body and Social Theory*, London: Sage.

Sidell, M. (1995) *Health in Old Age: Myth, Mystery and Management*, Buckingham: Open University.

Simpson, R. (1998) *Changing Families: An Ethnographic Approach to Divorce and Separation*, Oxford: Berg.

Skultans, V. (1974) *Intimacy and Ritual: A Study of Spiritualists, Mediums and Groups*, London: Routledge.

Slobodin, R. (1997) 'W.H.R. Rivers', cited in P. Barker, (1995) *The Ghost Road*, Harmondsworth: Penguin.

Stallybrass, P. and White, A. (1986) *The Politics and Poetics of Transgression*, London: Methuen.

Sudnow, D. (1967) *Passing On: The Social Organization of Dying*, New Jersey: Prentice-Hall.

Symon, A, and Cunningham, S. (1995) 'Handling premature neonates: a study using time lapse video', *Nursing Times*, 91 (17), 35–37.

Synott, A. (1992) 'Tomb, temple, machine and self: the social construction of the body', *British Journal of Sociology*, 43 (1), 79–110.

Terry, J. and Urla, J. (1995) *Deviant Bodies*, Bloomington and Indianapolis: Indiana University Press.

Thomas, K. (1971) *Religion and the Decline of Magic. Studies in Popular Beliefs in Sixteenth and Seventeenth Century England*, Harmondsworth: Penguin.

Tiryakian, E.A. (1974a) 'Preliminary considerations', in E.A. Tiryakian (ed.) *On the Margin of the Visible: Sociology, the Esoteric, and the Occult*, New York: John Wiley and Sons.

——(1974b) 'Towards the sociology of esoteric culture', in E.A. Tiryakian (ed.) *On the Margin of the Visible: Sociology, the Esoteric, and the Occult*, New York: John Wiley and Sons.

Townsend, C. (1998) *Vile Bodies: Photography and the Crisis of Looking*, Munich: Prestel-Verlag.

Truzzi, M. (1974) 'Definition and dimensions of the occult: towards a sociological perspective', in E.A. Tiryakian (ed.) *On the Margin of the Visible. Sociology, the Esoteric, and the Occult*, New York: John Wiley and Sons.

Turner, B.S. (1984) *The Body and Society*, Oxford: Basil Blackwell.

——(1987) *Medical Power and Social Knowledge*, London: Sage.

——(1992) *Regulating Bodies: Essays in Medical Sociology*, London: Routledge.

——(1995) 'Aging and identity: some reflections on the somatization of self', in M. Featherstone and A. Wernick (eds) *Images of Aging*, London: Routledge.

——(1996) *The Body and Society*, 2nd edition, London: Sage.

——(1998) Plenary paper given at the After the Body Conference, University of Manchester.

Turner, V. (1967) *The Forest of Symbols*, New York: Cornell University Press.

——(1974) *Dramas, Fields and Metaphors: Symbolic Action in Human Society*, Ithaca and London: Cornell University Press.

Van Gennep, A. ([1909] 1960) *The Rites of Passage*, Chicago: University of Chicago Press.

Vialles, N. (1994) *Animal to Edible*, Cambridge: Cambridge University Press.

Vitebsky, P. (1990) *Dialogues with the Dead: The Discussion of Mortality among the Sora of Central India*, Cambridge: Cambridge University Press.

——(1990) 'Piers Vitebsky', in R. Dinnage (ed.) *The Ruffian on the Stair*, Harmondsworth: Penguin.

Walter, T. (1990) *Funerals and How to Improve Them*, London: Hodder and Stoughton.

——(1996) 'A new model of grief', *Mortality*, 1 (1), 7–25.

Warner, M. 1995: 'The unbearable likeness of being, Part 2', *Tate: The Art Magazine*, Issue 7, Winter, 39–47.

——(1996) *The Inner Eye: Art Beyond the Visible*, National Touring Exhibitions, South Bank Centre.

Watson, J.L. (1982) 'Of flesh and bones: the management of death pollution in Cantonese society', in M. Bloch and J. Parry (eds), *Death and the Regeneration of Life*, Cambridge: Cambridge University Press.

Watt, T. (1994 [1991]) *Cheap Print and Popular Piety, 1550–1640*, Cambridge: Cambridge University Press.

Waugh, E. (1948) *The Loved One: An Anglo-American Tragedy*, London: Chapman and Hall.

Weedon, C. (1997) *Feminist Practice and Poststructuralist Theory*, Oxford: Blackwell Publishers.

Wilkinson, R. (1996) *Unhealthy Societies: the afflictions of inequality*, London: Routledge.

Williams, S. and Bendelow, G. (1998) 'In search of the "missing body"; pain, suffering and the (post) modern condition', in G. Scambler and P. Higgs (eds) *Modernity, Medicine and Health. Medical Sociology Towards 2000*, London: Routledge.

Williams, W.T. and Vallins, G.H. (eds) (1931) *Tennyson: Select Poems*, London, Methuen & Co Ltd.

Winterson, J. (1998) *The World and Other Places*, London: Jonathan Cape.

Worden, J. W. (1991) *Grief Counselling and Grief Therapy*, London: Routledge.

Young, J, (1997) 'To touch or not to touch?', *Modern Midwife*, 7 (6) 10–14.

Index